Beat Depression with St. John's Wort

Steven Bratman, M.D.

Prima Publishing

PRIMA PUBLISHING and colophon are trademarks of
Prima Communications, Inc.

Library of Congress Cataloging-in-Publication Data

Bratman, Steven.
Beat depression with St. John's wort / Steven Bratman.
p.   cm.
Includes index.
ISBN 0-7615-1297-7
1. Depression, Mental—Treatment.   2. Triadenum virginicum—Therapeutic use.
I. Title.
RC537.B747 1997
616.85'27061—dc21   97-34408
CIP

WARNING—DISCLAIMER

Prima Publishing has designed this book to provide information in regard to the subject matter covered. It is sold with the understanding that the publisher and the author are not liable for the misconception or misuse of information provided. Every effort has been made to make this book as complete and as accurate as possible. The purpose of this book is to educate. The author and Prima Publishing shall have neither liability nor responsibility to any person or entity with respect to any loss, damage, or injury caused or alleged to be caused directly or indirectly by the information contained in this book. The information presented herein is in no way intended as a substitute for medical counseling.

97 98 99 00 HH 10 9 8 7 6 5 4 3 2
Printed in the United States of America

How to Order

Single copies may be ordered from Prima Publishing, P.O. Box 1260BK, Rocklin, CA 95677; telephone (916) 632-4400. Quantity discounts are also available. On your letterhead, include information concerning the intended use of the books and the number of books you wish to purchase.

Visit us online at www.primapublishing.com

Contents

Dysthymia (mild to moderate depression). Chronic depressed mood, low energy, low self-esteem, poor concentration, difficulty making decisions, feelings of hopelessness, poor appetite (or overeating), insomnia (or excessive sleep). (Adapted from the *Diagnosis and Statistical Manual of Mental Disorders,* 4th edition, American Psychiatric Association, 1994.)

Note to the Reader

As a physician who practices a blend of alternative and conventional medicine, I have observed over the years that some alternative treatments really work, while others seem to be little more than wishful thinking. A large part of my task as a responsible professional is to sort through the innumerable treatment options and provide a clear view of which ones are truly helpful.

St. John's wort is one such useful treatment. Not only is the scientific data supporting it reasonably good, my clinical experiences and those of numerous other practitioners using the herb in daily practice have convinced me that St. John's wort is a splendid option for mild to moderate depression.

However, I am not putting it forward as a "miracle cure." Such hyperbole has become much too common in the alternative medicine literature. A treatment does not have to be "miraculous" to be thoroughly useful, and that is how I would like to present St. John's wort, when it is used in the context of a comprehensive approach to health care.

Introduction

Every year, millions of Americans seek treatment for depression, complaining of symptoms that interfere with their relationships, impair their work capacity, and deprive them of the full emotional experiences of life. For most of this century, psychotherapy has been the primary treatment for mild to moderate depression. However, psychotherapy is slow, expensive, and not always entirely successful. Many patients complain that they continue to experience depression even after years of otherwise useful psychotherapy.

Treatment for depression was revolutionized in the late 1980s with the production of Prozac, the first antidepressant drug truly appropriate for mild to moderate depression. Breaking all previous records for the use of antidepressants, Prozac quickly achieved what can only be described as cult status. "Tess," a patient made famous in Peter Kramer's *Listening to Prozac*, called herself Ms. Prozac, because she believed the drug gave her "charisma, courage, character, and social competency." So positive was Prozac's image for a time, it was widely called vitamin P.

Then a backlash set in; Prozac was found to be not nearly so side-effect-free as the manufacturer had suggested. A freedom-of-information request by psychiatrist Peter Breggin, author of *Talking Back to Prozac,* uncovered the fact that only 286 people, out of a reported 1,730, had completed the full side-effects studies prior to the release of Prozac. Real-life experiences revealed that Prozac (and similar drugs) frequently caused unpleasant symptoms ranging from merely annoying to absolutely intolerable.

Many patients on Prozac develop insomnia so severe that they must take a second drug at night to sleep. Women frequently complain of decreased libido and the inability to experience orgasm. Other common problems include anxiety, agitation, severe headaches, undesired weight loss, tremors, sweating, and short-term memory loss.

Furthermore, it has gradually become clear that Prozac seldom produces the magical results initially attributed to it and that even when good results are attained, progressively higher doses of the drug are often required to maintain them. The new antidepressants have thus proved to be less effective and far more problematic than initially believed. Nevertheless, Prozac is taken by millions of people. Although many who use the drug do experience significant relief, others turn to it primarily for its mystique and continue to take it more out of hope than out of actual results.

Interestingly, when the United States embraced Prozac, a completely different course was taken in Germany. Instead of turning to a new prescription drug, physicians there rediscovered an ancient treatment: the herb St. John's wort. Today, only 7 percent of the antidepressant prescriptions in Germany are written for Prozac; St. John's wort dominates the field.

It may seem surprising that an advanced technological society such as Germany's should place so great a reliance on an herb, but St. John's wort is a remarkable herb. Meaningful double-blind studies involving nearly 2,000 patients and published in reputable medical journals have shown that this traditional treatment for depression is safe and effective. Furthermore, in the clinical experience of many psychiatrists who prescribe it, St. John's wort is a better treatment for mild to moderate depression than drug therapy. It is often equally effective and almost always far gentler: the herb does not cause sexual dysfunction, insomnia, headaches, or anxiety.

As one patient said, "Taking St. John's wort was like filling a lake drop by drop. Almost without my being aware of it, the emptiness and hopelessness were gradually replaced by a quiet sense of calm. Taking Prozac was like being shot in the face with a firehose."

Gentler treatments are almost always worth trying before more disruptive ones. But the significance of St. John's wort's effectiveness is not limited to its gentleness. In terms of raw performance, St. John's wort sometimes outperforms all drugs available for treatment of depression. Later in this book I tell the story of a nursing-home patient who remained bedfast from depression despite successive treatment with Prozac, Zoloft, and Effexor. After two weeks' use of St. John's wort, he started walking about, interacting with staff and patients, and eating normally. This herb is no weakling; it can be a genuinely powerful force against depression.

Despite its remarkable combination of safety and effectiveness and its widespread use in Germany, St. John's wort was almost unknown in the United States until quite recently. This situation suddenly changed in early 1997, when strongly positive reporting in *Newsweek* and *The Washington Post*, and on *USA Weekend* and *20/20*, catapulted St. John's wort into public awareness. It now seems highly possible that America will soon follow Germany's lead and adopt this safe, natural substance as the primary prescription for mild to moderate depression.

Nonetheless, St. John's wort is not a panacea. It has its strengths and weaknesses like all other medical treatments, and this book objectively reports them. But for individuals who seek help for symptoms of depression and want a gentler, more natural approach than drugs, St. John's wort could indeed be a splendid option.

CHAPTER ONE

What Is St. John's Wort?

- Why it is called St. John's wort
- What is in it?
- How it was used historically

K nown officially as *Hypericum perforatum,* St. John's wort is a perennial herb of many branches and bright yellow flowers. It is fond of sun-exposed slopes and grows in dry grasslands, pastures, and sparse woods and alongside roadways. For its beautiful golden petals, St. John's wort is one of the most admired wild plants in Germany, but a more subtle artistic effect can be discovered on close inspection of the leaves. When held up to the light, a kind of watermark can be seen: translucent dots scattered in a pleasing pattern. It is these visual "perforations" that give it the species name *perforatum.*

Another distinguishing characteristic is numerous black dots on the sepals and petals of the flower. These release a red pigment when squeezed: the "blood" of Saint John, according to tradition.

Like all medicinal herbs, St. John's wort is a weed; in this case a powerful one. When it was brought over to the Americas by Europeans, *Hypericum* "went native" and became an invasive pest in the Pacific Northwest. It invaded pastures and ranchland, and threatened to become the kudzu of the north. Because cattle that devour large quantities of the herb can develop severe sunburn, local ranchers gave it the epithet Klamath Weed and undertook to stamp it out with poisons.

Herbicides failed, however, to make an impact. In 1946, an Australian beetle that possessed a voracious appetite for the herb was introduced as a kind of biological control: *Chrysolina quadregemina Rossi.* (Perhaps the beetles suffer from chronic depression, if one can imagine a depressed beetle.) *This* intervention was successful, and within ten years wild St. John's wort was reduced to 1 percent of its previous prevalence in Northern California. Ironically, these beetles may become a significant obstacle to the intentional U.S. cultivation of St. John's wort now underway.

Where Does the Name Come From?

A "wort" is simply a plant or an herb in Old English. There are many explanations for the traditional connection to

Saint John, but perhaps the simplest is that the herb flowers around the time of the feast of Saint John. Also, in Christian tradition, Saint John represents spiritual light coming to earth. The bright yellow color of the flowers may have thus clinched the connection by seeming to represent fragments of the sun brought close to the ground.

It is tempting to speculate further that the antidepressant effects of this herb may have provided another connection with Saint John. Spiritual light is the antithesis of depression. If you feel depressed, you might say that you feel "plunged into darkness," and when you recover, your friends might say that you've brightened up. Even advertisements for antidepressant drugs make use of this connection by, for example, showing a patient rising from bed and opening a brightly lit window.

Those who take St. John's wort often report that they feel a sensation like increased interior light. In the devout environment of the Middle Ages, this experience might well have been interpreted as the presence of a light-bearing saint.

The genus name *Hypericum* also has its meaningful history. According to the noted herbalist Christopher Hobbs, an older name for the genus was *Hyperikon,* deriving from the combination of the words *hyper* (above) and *eikon* (a figure with supernatural characteristics). Hobbs relates this derivation to the traditional use of St. John's wort as a protection against demons, witches, and other supernatural beings. Since our ancestors attributed symptoms of depression to the influence of demonic forces, could it be that the name *Hypericum* indicates that St. John's wort was known to be effective for depression?

What Is in St. John's Wort?

If the crushed flowers of St. John's wort are steeped in vegetable oil for several weeks, the liquid takes on deep red tones that fluoresce in sunlight. The fluorescent constituent is a chemical named *hypericin,* and it is this substance that is most commonly cited as the herb's active ingredient. However, this has not been conclusively proved. Like all herbs, St. John's wort contains innumerable organic chemicals in varying concentrations. It is perfectly possible that another ingredient, or combination of ingredients, is actually responsible for the antidepressant effect.

An abbreviated list of the constituents of St. John's wort includes: flavonols, flavanones, coumarins, xanthones, phenolic carboxylic acids, carotenoids, phytosterols, n-alkanols, n-alkanes, sequiterpenes, monoterpenes, and a great variety of dianthrones (of which hypericin is only one member). More on what is known about the chemical basis of St. John's wort's mood-elevating properties is discussed in a later chapter.

What Was It Used for Historically?

From the times of the ancient Greeks, plants of the genus *Hypericum* have been used for a variety of medicinal purposes, such as healing burns and other skin injuries, counteracting snake bite, treating ulcers, and improving the flow of urine. St. John's wort was used in Celtic religious practices in England, and subsequently the herb took on an unofficial spiritual significance among Christians. European herbalists frequently called it *Fuga daemonum,* in reference to widespread belief that St. John's wort could drive away demons.

Thus, again we return to the spiritual connotations of St. John's wort. It is almost irresistible to hypothesize that the presumed supernatural powers of St. John's wort stemmed from a primeval appreciation of its antidepressant characteristics. If you lived in the Middle Ages and your neighbor was unaccountably sad, troubled by guilt, and crippled by anxiety, you would very likely come to believe that he or she was afflicted by demons. If your neighbor then started to drink a daily brew of St. John's wort tea and subsequently recovered from this "demonic possession," you probably couldn't fail to assign magical potency to the herb. It would not be very long before you might feel inspired to use the herb as a symbolic protection, perhaps by wearing it about your neck. An old poem shows this reverence clearly:

> *St. John's Wort doth charm all the witches away,*
> *If gathered at midnight on the saint's holy day.*
> *And devils and witches have no power to harm*
> *Those that do gather the plant for a charm.*

> —from Christopher Hobbs,
> *HerbalGram* no. 18/19, pp. 25–26, 1989

If we in modern times were similarly inclined, I could easily imagine people wearing a necklace of Prozac pills to ward off gloomy thoughts. While I have never heard of anyone taking quite that course, it is not at all unusual for patients on Prozac to use the drug as a kind of mental amulet. Whenever they suffer rejection or another experience likely to provoke depression they remind themselves that they are "under the protection of Prozac" and needn't fear emotional collapse. This positive self-suggestion is quite sensible, but it amounts to a talismanic use of the drug. In this respect we are no different from our medieval ancestors who felt reassured by the presence of St. John's wort, whether internally or externally.

When scientific medicine began to predominate, references to the psychological effects of St. John's wort started to take a more modern turn. Literature from around the turn of the twentieth century reports the herb to be useful for nervous imbalances, hysteria, and depression, putting it in the category of "nervine" or "nerve tonic." In recent decades, the development of chemical antidepressants has inspired scientists who are aware of this herbal tradition to look for similar properties in St. John's wort.

Early studies focused on determining whether the constituents of St. John's wort functioned similarly to a class of antidepressants known as MAO inhibitors. Later research focused on a serotonin connection, as discussed in chapter 5. At the same time, formal trials were begun to determine the clinical effectiveness of St. John's wort in the treatment of depression. The results were so positive that by 1988 St. John's wort was officially approved as an antidepressant drug in Germany.

During the period of explosive growth of Prozac use in the United States, St. John's wort became the dominant antidepressant treatment in Germany and was soon widely used in other European countries as well. In 1993, the latest year for which records are available, German physicians issued more than 2.7 million prescriptions for St. John's wort.

The culture of conventional medicine in Europe is rather receptive to herbal treatment. In the United States, however, acceptance of St. John's wort as a scientifically validated treatment for depression was delayed by the prejudice against herbal medicine that characterizes the U.S. medical culture. The highly respected naturopathic physician and author Michael Murray was one of several responsible authorities who attempted to bring forward in the United States the European experience with St. John's wort, but it was not until 1997 that this effort bore fruit. St. John's wort is now poised for take-off here as a substitute for drug therapy.

But before discussing how this herb can be used for depression, I must interpose a brief discussion of depression itself.

CHAPTER TWO

The Symptoms of Depression

- Mild to moderate versus major
- Depressed mood
- Numbness
- Irritability
- Sleep disturbances
- Low energy
- Low self-esteem
- Poor concentration or difficulty making decisions
- Feelings of hopelessness
- Eating disorders
- Emptiness
- Anxiety
- Guilt
- Obsession with body symptoms
- Difficulty managing stress
- Hidden forms of depression
- Excessive shyness
- Oversensitivity to rejection
- Lack of assertiveness
- Inability to take risks

Mild to Moderate Versus Major

To most people, the term *depression* indicates a dampened mood and pervasive unhappiness. However, the medical profession generally reserves that term for the catastrophic state of major depression. For what the public calls mild to moderate depression, doctors frequently use the technical term *dysthymia*.

Thus to have been medically accurate this book could have been titled *Beat Dysthymia with St. John's Wort,* but only medical professionals would have known what was meant. Throughout this book *depression* is used to mean mild to moderate depression, unless otherwise specified.

It is important to settle this semantics question at the outset because St. John's wort is an appropriate treatment only for mild to moderate depression. It should not be used for severe major depressive conditions. In order to make the difference between the two conditions clear, I would like to begin by describing major depression.

According to author William Styron (quoted in *On the Edge of Darkness* [Dell, 1995], by Kathy Cronkite) "it's sadness that has become intensified into excruciating pain." Along with unremitting unhappiness comes paralyzing self-judgment, obsessive guilty rumination, numbness, loss of interest in normal activities, incapacity to deal with life, and recurrent thoughts of death by suicide. The sufferer's life collapses, and suicide becomes an imminent possibility. There are physical symptoms in major depression, as well, including slowed movements, markedly delayed responses to questions, and drawn-out speech. Occasional episodes of frantic activity may arise briefly, only to subside back into leaden slowness.

One might say that in major depression the emotional structure of the brain freezes into a pattern of misery. It cannot be shaken by any ordinary external event because the computer, so to speak, is locked up. Indeed, one of the earliest successful treatments for major depression was shock therapy, a technique that can be compared to the rebooting of a computer.

However, when shock treatment first came out, it was drastically overused and barbarically applied, and so fell into disrepute. Antidepressant drugs were the next breakthrough treatment. Practically any pharmaceutical antidepressant has the capacity to lift a patient out of major depression, and for this purpose, drugs are indispensable and may even be lifesaving.

As previously mentioned, St. John's wort is not an appropriate treatment for major depression. However, when most people say "I'm depressed" they're probably referring to something much less catastrophic. Life may be difficult, but it isn't impossible. Perhaps you feel constantly fatigued, but you succeed in getting out of bed; and though you may feel unhappy, you're not ready to end it all. It is for this much more common type of depression that St. John's wort is useful, and perhaps more appropriate than drug treatment.

Drugs were originally invented for major depression. However, following the advent of Prozac, it became popular to prescribe antidepressants for mild to moderate depression as well. But because there are so many side effects with such drugs, this may be overkill.

In cases of major depression, it is reasonable to put up with a few side effects. After all, the alternative could be suicide. When depression is only mild to moderate, however, it isn't quite so reasonable to take a drug that can cause anxiety, severe insomnia or loss of the ability to achieve an orgasm. St. John's wort is often a much better option.

In the remainder of this chapter, the various symptoms of mild to moderate depression are explored. The effectiveness of treatment by drugs, St. John's wort, and psychotherapy is also sketched briefly, while subsequent chapters delve further into each of these treatment options.

Depressed Mood

For many people, depression connotes sadness, gloom, and a sense of pervading melancholy. Feelings of unhappiness float just beneath the surface, ready to attach themselves to any outward event and make you say to yourself, "I told you so! You have every reason to feel miserable." If you experience this kind of depression you may burst into tears on the slightest provocation, and when you look at the future it may seem to hold mostly the promise of failure. As one patient said to me, "It used to be I could look at my children and feel proud. Now I keep thinking how I'm failing them, and how they'll probably turn out all messed up, like me."

These symptoms are similar to those of major depression, but milder. Thoughts of suicide may flit by, but you have no real inclination to act on them. Crying spells almost always occur for a reason, unlike the almost continuous, unexplainable crying of major depression. Finally, you have both good and bad days, and happiness usually manages to break through the unhappiness at least once or twice a day.

A patient whom I shall call Ann is a good example of someone experiencing this form of depression. To all outward appearances she was perfectly well adjusted. She had a happy family and a good job, and only those who knew her well knew that anything was wrong.

But one day Ann confessed her inner feelings to her doctor. "I'm just forcing a smile all day," she said. "It's an act I have to keep up from morning to night. Inside, I feel like I've just been to a funeral. I don't know why."

Although Ann went to counselors and therapists for years and had thoroughly worked through the few childhood traumas that could be identified, the sadness just wouldn't go away. When her doctor suggested antidepressants, Ann was reluctant at first. "I don't want to be dependent on a drug," she'd said. But when she finally did take the antidepressant Zoloft, she was amazed by the results. "Nothing changed about me except that I didn't feel sad anymore. It was like someone carved away my misery with a knife. I felt bright inside, and didn't have to fake my smile."

Apparently, Ann is one of those people for whom depression is primarily from a biochemical cause. Psychotherapy had been useful, but it couldn't touch her chronically depressed mood. Drug therapy was a revelation.

Ann soon became a walking advertisement for Zoloft. She told all her friends about how much it had helped her, and, for a brief period, even considered writing a book about it. But within a month she discovered that there was a price to pay for her improvement—in side effects.

She developed diarrhea, headaches, and mild insomnia. But she could live with those. What Ann could not tolerate was anorgasmia: the complete inability to have an orgasm. She had no trouble becoming aroused, but she "felt like a train all revved up with nowhere to go." Before Zoloft, her sex life had been free from problems. She decided this symptom was intolerable.

She also hated the feeling of being on a drug. "I always feel like there's something foreign in my system, something chemical," she explained. For these two reasons Ann quit taking Zoloft after a couple of months. Unfortunately, she started to feel sad again almost immediately. "It was like my insides just drained away. The melancholy came right back like before."

Her psychiatrist suggested the drug Serzone, an antidepressant that typically does not interfere with orgasm. Unfortunately, "Serzone made me into a walking zombie." As a third try, Prozac was prescribed but caused terrific insomnia. "I finally decided I'd rather be depressed than put up with all these disgusting side effects," she said when she came to me.

It seemed that Ann was a perfect candidate for St. John's wort. Although she was depressed, she wasn't paralyzed by her depression. Her sadness was uncomfortable, but it wasn't unbearable pain; and she never felt so bad that she would consider suicide. Thus, Ann fit the picture of mild to moderate depression.

It took about six weeks for St. John's wort to achieve full effect. "It came on gently and gradually," Ann said. "The sadness didn't shut off all at once like on Zoloft, but it gradually evaporated. I didn't have any side effects, either." What's more, Ann enjoyed the feeling of taking a natural herb instead of a chemical.

Of course, testimonials such as this one are of no scientific value. One success says nothing about general effectiveness, and, indeed, St. John's wort doesn't always work as well as it did for Ann. (Drugs don't always work so well either!) The formal research that scientifically evaluates St. John's wort's effectiveness is explored in chapters 5 snd 7.

Numbness

Gloom and sadness aren't the only moods associated with depression. For some people, dullness, numbness, and apathy predominate. These forms of depression make it difficult to get very excited about anything, either good or bad. Nothing seems to matter very much at all. "I don't really care if I go out on a date or stay home," one patient said. "It's all the same to me."

In mild to moderate depression, this state of numbness isn't absolute. Desires percolate beneath the surface, such as wanting to go out on a date, only they seem like too much trouble. This is a milder symptom than what occurs with major depression, where desires seem dead and buried. But the relative apathy of mild to moderate depression is quite enough to destroy initiative and paralyze activity. As one patient explained, "I can only be bothered to do what I have to do. Occasionally, I do go out for fun, but only when it all falls together by itself."

Antidepressants can be quite successful with this form of depression. Caring and interest may come back again, but some patients complain that there is an artificial quality to their renewed involvement with life. As one patient said, "I go out dancing now but sometimes it feels like it's the Prozac dancing instead of me." St. John's wort may be preferable because it can increase the ability to feel without taking over.

Irritability

Depressed mood and numbness are immediately recognizable as types of depression. However, there is another type that may go unrecognized, even by professionals. This is unusual irritability, a common dominant mood in depressed children and adolescents.

Everyone is irritable sometimes (especially teenagers!). Not enough sleep, a rushed schedule, too many responsibilities, or simply a "bad day" can cause irritability in the best of us. But the irritability of hidden depression has a quality that psychologists call "overdetermined." It seems to have a life of its own, regardless of whether there are any contributing circumstances that might reasonably be expected to cause it.

The idea that irritability can mask depression is not new, but recent evidence supporting it has come through "listening to antidepressants," as Peter Kramer evocatively describes this increasingly influential process in psychiatry.

Physicians have observed that when hyperirritable people take antidepressants, they frequently become much calmer. However, antidepressants are not tranquilizers and do not universally produce a sense of calm. The calming effect is remarkably specific to a certain kind of irritability, which has led to thinking that that kind of irritability is really depression in disguise.

This reasoning has been criticized as being somewhat circular. Nonetheless, the discovery that hyperirritability often responds to antidepressant treatment has been a great boon to many children and their families. Clinically speaking, St. John's wort is often just as effective as medications.

And for children, there is one great advantage to using the herb instead of a drug. Taking a drug seems to send the message "you're sick." Since children respond readily to symbolism, after taking drugs for a year or more they may internalize that message and view themselves as basically broken.

An herbal treatment can be honestly presented as a kind of food. As one psychiatrist said to his ten-year-old patient, "This herb feeds your patience. It makes it stronger." Thinking of yourself as in need of nourishment feels a lot better than believing that you are broken and need to be fixed by taking a drug. It creates a much better self-image.

With adolescents, the problem is slightly different. If you tell a teenager that a drug will cure his or her depression, this suggests that drugs are good options for altering mood. The leap from taking a prescription drug to taking an illegal drug may not seem very far. If you give the teenager an herb instead, with its connotations of being a natural, healthful treatment, it is possible to maintain the separation from taking unhealthy illegal drugs.

Sleep Disturbances

Depression can cause either insomnia or the need for excessive sleep. When the prevailing symptom is insomnia, it is a special kind of insomnia: early morning awakening. You may be able to fall asleep well enough, but somewhere between three and five in the morning you find yourself suddenly wide awake. This puts you in an awkward situation. If you simply get up and get out of bed, you'll feel terrible the rest of the day: exhausted, headachy, and unable to concentrate. If you stay in bed, however, you'll just toss and turn and probably start worrying about something.

Antidepressants can benefit sleep in one of two ways. The older antidepressants, such as amitriptylline and trazadone, cause drowsiness directly and make pretty good sleeping pills. Unfortunately, they can also produce a drugged feeling round the clock. Most of them can also cause dramatic weight gain.

The newer antidepressants are not sleeping pills. In fact, many create a stimulating effect that can at first make insomnia much worse. Sleeping only begins to improve once the full antidepressant effect sets in, which may take as long as four to six weeks. Apparently, the disturbances of brain chemicals that occur in depression also cause early morning awakening. When a better balance is restored through successful drug treatment, sleep improves at the same time.

This effect isn't a sure thing, however. The stimulating side effects of the new antidepressants can be so strong that the net result is to make insomnia far worse. Frequently those individuals for whom insomnia is a part of their depression find that they must take two antidepressants: one to wake up and another to go to sleep.

For many patients, this two-drug approach doesn't feel right. As one patient said to me, "It's like being on uppers and downers. I started to think I was Bob Fosse in *All That Jazz.*" St. John's wort is a wonderful option for patients with depression-induced insomnia because it relieves depression without causing either excessive wakefulness or daytime drowsiness.

When the prevailing symptom of depression is excessive sleepiness, different considerations apply. Peter was a patient of mine who when depressed went to bed as early as seven in the evening and would still resent the alarm clock when it woke him at eight the following morning. He found that Prozac cured his excessive sleeping in short order, but the effect was too dramatic. He could only sleep four hours a night. Peter ultimately found that he preferred the gentler energizing effects of St. John's wort.

Low Energy or Fatigue

Many patients visit the doctor's office for the sole complaint of fatigue. Unfortunately, a partial list of the medical diseases that can cause fatigue would fill at least a page. Attempting a diagnosis can involve a great number of tests, and in the end, there may still be no diagnosis.

In many cases, the sensation of fatigue may be due to problems in the fine-tuning of the body too subtle for medicine to identify. Sometimes the underlying cause of tiredness, however, is depression. There is no doubt of the converse: depression can cause a pervading sense of low energy.

Several patients who seem to be particularly perceptive about their own sensations have told me that the fatigue of depression has a unique character. "It seems to have its roots in my soul," one said. "I'm weary like I've just been through a battle." Another patient explained it this way: "Children have a connection to heaven that makes them bounce, and, although it gradually fades, a healthy grown-up shouldn't have lost it all. But I have no bounce. I have to use my will when love should be enough."

There may be a brief burst of energy in the morning or evening, but patients with depression-induced fatigue drag through most of the day. Even play may come to feel like work. Again, this symptom is milder with dysthymia than with major depression, where the energy loss is so profound it can mimic severe physical illness. The fatigue of mild to moderate depression is unpleasant and debilitating, but it is only occasionally overwhelming.

When it is a symptom of depression, fatigue typically responds very well to the Prozac class of drugs. But St. John's wort is an excellent option. One of the most common statements I hear from patients who take this herb is that they feel energized. Furthermore, this energizing effect rises slowly and gradually, without the jaggedness and edginess so common with antidepressant therapy.

Low Self-Esteem

Patients who are depressed typically possess a low opinion of their own value. A critical voice runs continually in their minds, providing an unwanted commentary on everything they do. "There you go, blowing it as usual. Why bother trying to do that; you'll fail. Don't talk to *them;* why would they be interested in you? You're a nobody." This constant disparagement can be very destructive.

One of the worst characteristics of low self-esteem is that it is self-reinforcing. For example, if I believe that I cannot possibly get a good job, I won't even bother applying, or if I do apply, I'll convey by word and body language that no sensible employer would ever want to hire me. Unless an employer takes me on out of a sense of charity, I'll probably end up with jobs that I am overqualified for or that no one else wants to take. The inner critic will then take my misfortune for an opportunity. "See? You're no good," it will say. "Look at the kind of work you have to do. It just goes to show how worthless you are."

This is really very unfair, because it was the inner critic itself that caused the problem in the first place. But inner critics are seldom fair. Although they frequently pretend to have our best interest at heart ("I'm only telling you this for your own good"), it's all a sham. Sometimes, the inner critic seems to have no greater aim than to cause unhappiness.

Low self-esteem interferes with relationships just as much as with jobs. As one patient said to me, "I don't bother trying to go out with men I really like, because they seem out of reach. The way I feel you'd think this was the 1800s and I was a peasant in love with an aristocrat. The good ones seem 'above me' or 'out of my league.' It isn't logical, but that's how it goes. So I pursue guys that I really don't like. I don't seem to think I'm good enough unless the guy's a low-life."

In many cases, low self-esteem is brought on by problems in childhood. The inner critic is often a carbon copy of parents or siblings who used constant shaming as a tool. A good psychotherapist can help us understand the origin of the inner critic, separate ourselves from its voice, and provide an alternative stream of positive mental commentary. But this approach isn't always completely successful. Sometimes, it seems that brain chemicals become so poisoned that no amount of positive self-encouragement can make a difference.

It is in this condition that antidepressant therapy can be particularly helpful. Drugs seem to push the inner critic into the background, where it can be managed more easily. As one patient said to me, "The critical voice is still there, but it's not right in my face. It's somewhere across the room now. I don't have to listen to it." By elevating mood, St. John's wort can sometimes provide the same benefit.

Poor Concentration or Difficulty Making Decisions

Depression can make simple tasks and decision making much more difficult. It's like there's an undertow. The constant drag of depression interferes with your thinking processes. You mix up simple instructions, go on Thursday to a Friday appointment, and go to the store and can't remember why. You can't decide whether to buy the wool sweater or the cotton sweater, because your inner critic gets in the way and politely informs you that whatever you decide will be wrong.

Treatment for depression by any proven method often alleviates this symptom. When depression is no longer grumbling away in the depths, your mind breaks free from its troubling preoccupation and can then get down to business. One patient said to me, "When I got over being depressed it seemed like my IQ jumped twenty points."

Unfortunately, antidepressant drugs can cause mental confusion, memory loss, and a sense of disorientation as direct side effects. Common descriptions include: "I feel scatterbrained," "I can't remember anything," and "Half the time I don't even know where I am." In such cases, St. John's wort may be a better choice. It doesn't seem to have any adverse mental effects, so its benefits for depression are not counteracted by drug-induced confusion.

Feelings of Hopelessness

Hope is one of the most universal of human needs, but in depression it's severely strained. Under normal circumstances, each morning brings some optimism. No matter how dark the future seemed last night, when the sun comes up, more options seem possible than you previously thought. But depression can take away much of this natural rejuvenation. The morning may bring with it no more enthusiasm than the night before, and you may have to get by on mere dogged persistence.

While patients with major depression frequently lose all hope and turn to suicide, in the mild to moderate depression discussed here there is enough hope to get by. However, there is not as much as there should be. One of the first signs of improving depression is a renewed sense of possibilities in life. Any successful treatment for depression can produce this positive result, whether psychotherapy, antidepressant drugs, or St. John's wort.

Eating Disorders

As on sleeping habits, the effect of depression on eating habits can go two ways. Some people overeat to compensate for their unhappiness, while others lose interest in food.

The most common of these possibilities is the familiar eating-for-comfort that can also occur without accompanying depression. When depression is involved, recovery from it will tend to normalize eating habits. However, most of the antidepressants in common use prior to Prozac often directly cause weight gain and an increase in appetite. Amitriptylline is one of the worst; weight increases of over sixty pounds are not uncommon during treatment with this somewhat outdated medication.

Drugs in the Prozac family are much better in this regard. Not only do they not cause weight gain as a side effect; in many cases they directly promote weight loss. This effect is discussed in *Safer Than Phen-fen* (Prima, 1997), by Michael Anchors. It doesn't appear likely that the use of St. John's wort will provide any similar benefit with regard to weight loss, other than through its effect on depression.

But when the eating disturbance caused by depression is loss of interest in food, Prozac-type drugs can be an obstacle, while St. John's wort, with its lack of side effects, may help to restore appetite more effectively.

Emptiness

Depression often brings with it a kind of inner emptiness or hollowness. All people experience a sense of emptiness from time to time, but depression amplifies this normal human experience. As one patient said, "I feel if someone could see inside me they'd find that there's not much there."

Of course, this sensation is an illusion. Every human being is a complex, amazing creature, a walking universe of thoughts, feelings, and talents. But depression can make it very difficult to feel your own richness. If depressed, even when others find you charming and interesting, you may wonder what they see in you, if you let yourself recognize their appreciation at all.

One of the first signs of recovery from depression is a feeling of being more filled up inside. Any of the many treatments for depression can help produce this result.

Anxiety

Anxiety can be a disease all in its own right, but it frequently accompanies depression. Of course, life is anxiety provoking in general. When anxiety becomes excessive, or when it detaches itself from real concerns and floats through your mental life like an ever-present cloud, that is when it is a real problem. One patient described the feeling like this: "I'm always sure disaster is just around the corner." Depression magnifies anxiety by decreasing the natural defenses against it.

In some cases anxiety gives rise to panic attacks. These can produce such severe heart pounding, chest pressure, and sense of impending doom that they may be confused with symptoms of a heart attack.

Antidepressants have proved to be useful treatments for anxiety. However, it is their long-term antidepressant effect that relieves symptoms. In the short term, most of the newer antidepressants have a disturbing potential to increase anxiety. Patients who are already anxious seldom appreciate being told that a medication may make them feel worse for the first month or so. St. John's wort, with its virtual absence of side effects, can be a very useful alternate choice.

Guilt

The actor and director Woody Allen has made an art of guilt, but the symptoms he presents in exaggerated forms are immediately recognizable to anyone who suffers from depression. That nagging sense that you've done something wrong, obsession with past errors, and overscrupulous concern about hurting someone's feelings: all of these go along with depression almost as inevitably as depressed mood.

Like so many symptoms of depression, guilt in itself is not an illness. If we never felt guilt (or the related emotion shame) we would all behave as selfishly as two-year-olds. But in depression, guilt is overdetermined. Guilt over specific events seems almost an excuse. Rather, the guilt is free floating, waiting for an event to which it can attach. Guilt feelings usually, but not always, retreat to manageable levels as depression is resolved. St. John's wort may be as helpful here as chemical antidepressants.

Obsession with Body Symptoms

Many people who are depressed find that they spend altogether too much time focusing on body symptoms. A mild spell of constipation, a headache, or a stiff neck can take on significance all out of proportion to the actual discomfort. There are many factors behind this commonly observed phenomenon. Because depression limits interest in our external lives, internal phenomena begin to loom larger. When depressed, we also have fewer inner resources to cope with discomfort and therefore succumb more easily. In addition, the anxiety associated with depression can give rise to terrible fantasies of cancer and imminent death, causing our minds to dwell on symptoms and our imaginations to amplify them.

Furthermore, there seems to be a direct relationship between depression and pain, as if the brain chemicals involved in each are similar. Many patients with chronic pain experience a marked improvement after starting antidepressant therapy. Unfortunately, medical doctors sometimes turn this observation around and make a weapon of it. For example, if a patient doesn't recover from a whiplash injury in the time the doctor expects, the physician may use what he knows about depression to shift blame. Too many patients are told, "You don't have any pain; you're just depressed."

This is an unfortunate distortion of the real situation. Just because depression amplifies discomfort doesn't mean the pain is "all in your head," and I sincerely wish doctors would quit using that expression. It is demeaning, hurtful, and ultimately useless.

Nonetheless, antidepressant medication can be quite helpful in dealing with pain. Whether the effect is due to changing brain chemicals, or simply to the fact that with an elevated mood it's easier to deal with pain, such treatment can often help. St. John's wort is a real option here.

Difficulty Managing Stress

Few of us handle stress particularly well, but depression turns "difficult" into "almost impossible." The ordinary stresses of daily life can easily overwhelm someone who is also dealing with depression.

On reflection, this shouldn't be surprising. When you suffer from depression, part of your brain is always busy processing guilt feelings, scanning for rejection, and expecting the worst. Have you ever used a computer that's trying to perform two tasks at the same time, such as print a document while running another program? The main program may slow to a crawl because the computer has to use part of its "brain" to concentrate on printing. Something similar happens when you are depressed. You lack the resources to deal with life's stresses successfully because much of your brain is occupied elsewhere.

In such a situation, successful treatment of depression by any route may make managing stress easier. As one patient said, "After I started to take St. John's wort, I found that I could deal much more patiently with my nagging boss and whining children."

Hidden Forms of Depression

Besides the direct symptoms of depression presented, there are several personality traits that psychologists have begun to suspect might represent depression in disguise. This impression has developed as a consequence of "listening to Prozac," as mentioned in my description of irritability. Through observing certain personality traits diminishing after starting Prozac, some physicians have concluded that those traits could actually be forms of depression.

It is also possible, however, that an underlying depression is simply exacerbating a personality trait that exists for other reasons. When the depression diminishes, other parts of the personality can come to the fore.

The argument against this simple viewpoint is that in perhaps one in twenty cases, Prozac seems to provide a benefit beyond what would be expected from simple lifting of depression. Speculation is rife that certain personality characteristics are identical to depression in some biochemical sense.

Not everyone agrees. It is possible that what we are seeing in those anecdotes is not really a curing of depression, but an incidental alterating of brain chemistry that happens to produce a pleasant result. After all, cocaine and alcohol can reduce shyness. In other words, personality changes may be a lucky side effect of Prozac.

But Prozac can cause unlucky side effects too. Some people experience negative personality changes on Prozac, such as increased aggression, irritability, and explosive anger. Furthermore, the positive personality-changing effects of Prozac may require continually increasing doses, presenting further similarity to cocaine and alcohol.

This subject is a discussion in progress. But one fact isn't controversial: depression can certainly contribute to personality difficulties of any kind, especially the ones listed below.

Excessive Shyness

A depressed person has to battle inner voices making such unpleasant comments as "You're unattractive," "You sound stupid," and "No one would want to listen to you." Who wouldn't be shy under those circumstances? One response to such inner voices is to avoid situations that trigger them.

I remember one young woman in her twenties who was so shy she didn't dare take a job that required contact with the public. What Lisa really wanted to do was become a veterinarian, because she loved animals, but she knew she couldn't face the interview process necessary to get into school. She took a low-paying job as an assistant bookkeeper instead, because it allowed her to hide.

Years of psychotherapy had helped Lisa understand why she felt this way, but it was only when she took Prozac that she could overcome her fears. She still had to work at it, but drug treatment was a useful and important step forward for her.

Unfortunately, along with its boost, Prozac gave her diarrhea, heart palpitations, and headaches. Other antidepressants caused similarly intolerable side effects. When she finally tried St. John's wort Lisa found an antidepressant medication she could live with. With the help of St. John's wort and the skills she had learned in psychotherapy she found herself equal to the task of overcoming her fears.

Oversensitivity to Rejection

Extreme sensitivity to rejection and other emotionally unpleasant experiences may also represent a covert form of depression in some people. Of course, none of us likes to be rejected, but in order to have a social life, we find it necessary to take that risk. Only by staying home alone all of the time can we completely eliminate the possibility that someone may express dislike for our company.

For some people, however, staying at home all of the time sounds pretty good. You may be so sensitive to rejection that you would rather face loneliness and social isolation than run any risk of experiencing what could be a cata-strophically painful event.

I remember a forty-five-year-old patient who had re-mained single all of his life because at the first hint of dis-pleasure from a potential partner he wanted to run. As he described it, "I just don't have enough of myself inside me to handle rejection. If I get a hint that a woman is going to show she doesn't like me, I start to feel like I don't exist. When I actually do get rejected it hurts worse than a broken bone. I feel like I'm dying."

Rejection isn't the only form of unpleasant emotional experience that can cause depressed people to "crash." Mild criticism from a bank teller, a bad grade in school, or even a rude honk in traffic can be enough to provoke a painful and prolonged response in those who are excessively thin-skinned. Very likely, depression plays a role for many people who suffer from these extreme emotional reactions, and any proven treatment for depression will provide at least some relief.

Lack of Assertiveness

Depression can also get in the way of assertiveness. As one patient said to me, "How can I stand up for myself when I think I'm nobody?" She would act like a doormat most of the time and then suddenly explode with resentment.

Psychologists speak of finding the midway point be-tween aggression and passivity. As depression improves, this point of healthy assertiveness may become much easier to achieve. Psychotherapy is probably the most helpful treat-ment here, but occasionally Prozac seems to spectacularly increase assertiveness all by itself. I have not heard any reports of similarly dramatic results produced by St. John's wort.

Inability to Take Risks

Life involves numerous risks. Unless we are willing to run the risk of failing we can't succeed: a cliché that is nonetheless true. But some people find it very difficult to take any risks at all. They feel compelled to choose the most cautious course at every decision point in life. Of course, cautiousness is not a disease. The continuum that goes from excessive caution to excessive risk taking includes a wide spectrum that is normal.

But some people are so cautious that it is more of a problem than a simple personality trait. Or, they may feel a strong desire to take more risks but feel an inner compulsion against it. This excessive cautiousness may very well be a form of depression.

It isn't difficult to understand how a general sense of gloominess and negativity would raise the stakes in any form of risky behavior. Overcautiousness may thus respond well to antidepressant treatment, whether with drugs or St. John's wort. Psychotherapy is usually essential as well.

There are many more possible manifestations and variations to the symptoms of depression. But this brief introduction allows us to turn to theories of what causes depression.

CHAPTER THREE

What Causes Depression?

- Software versus hardware
- Ancient theories
- The four humors
- The insights of psychotherapy
- The rise of the amine hypothesis
- Flaws in the amine hypothesis
- The big picture

There is no one cause for depression. Actually, no complex problem has a single cause or cure, whether it's the high divorce rate in the United States or the conflicts in the Middle East. Attempts throughout history to understand depression have led to a variety of theories and suggested treatments. These approaches can be understood, however, as a swing back and forth between two basic stances: viewing depression as a problem either in the "software" or in the "hardware" of the brain.

Computers require both software and hardware to run effectively. Software theories of depression look to the thoughts and feelings produced by actions, intentions, and experience, whereas hardware theories focus on the physical structures of the brain and body themselves. In reality, both approaches have their validity and enduring significance.

Ancient Theories of Depression

Perhaps the earliest "software" explanation for depression invoked the influence of deities or spirits. In her wonderful biography of Alexander the Great, *Fire from Heaven,* author Mary Renault shows how ancient Greeks attributed their moods to the active intervention of their gods. When Alexander felt confidence and power, he assumed that Hercules was infusing his soul with divine energy; but when he fell into despondency, he presumed that his actions had offended one or another of the deities he believed ruled his life.

Like all theories, this explanation for depression led to certain lines of "treatment." An ancient Greek afflicted with prolonged despondency might very well have felt impelled to make a sacrifice to the gods, consult with the Oracle at Delphi, or make a change in plans or behavior. Thus, religious action may be considered one of the earliest treatments for depression, and there is no doubt that it frequently succeeds, even today. Modern worshippers may experience a profound uplifting of the spirit after engaging in prayer or other religious rituals. But this was not the only Greek attitude toward depression.

The Four Humors

The ancient Greeks had another perspective on depression as well, one that falls into the "hardware" category. This perspective came out of the dominant scientific approach to medicine of the day, the theory of humors. Although it sounds preposterous now, the humor theory of medicine was the foundation of Hippocrates' approach to healing, and it continued to influence the practice of medicine up through the nineteenth century.

According to this theory, four "humors" constantly flow through the body. Hippocrates called them yellow bile, blood, phlegm, and black bile. A state of balance among these subtle substances is supposed to produce health, while a loss of balance initiates disease. In a state of perfect balance of the humors, perfect equanimity and health would result.

An excess of a particular humor was believed to produce not only physical illness but also certain characteristic emotional tendencies or temperaments. Respectively, these were described as choleric (angry), sanguine (emotional), phlegmatic (slow to respond), and melancholic (sad). Each of these names has its origin in the associated humor. For example, *melancholy* literally means black bile, because the Greek words for black and bile are *melan* and *cholia*.

Thus, in the humor system of illness, depression is a result of too much black bile. Appropriate treatment for depression under this system would aim not so much at curing the symptoms of depression but at reducing the level of black bile to normal, perhaps raising the other humors at the same time.

The humoral approach to health was still a dominant influence on conventional medicine in nineteenth-century Europe and America. Doctors of that day used leeching to "remove heat from the blood." And when a physician of the nineteenth century recommended a commonsense treatment for depression, such as spending more time outdoors, taking a vacation, or moving to a different climate, he would couch this advice in terms of its good effect on the humors.

But competing theories of depression that fit more into the software category also flourished, and one of them, the psychological approach, eventually came to dominate.

Back to Software

In medieval Europe, depression was often attributed to the influence of demonic forces. These supernatural powers were believed capable of entering a human being and producing unexplainable moods and evil actions. One remedy for this was prayer and fasting, another was exorcism, and in the popular mind at least, St. John's wort was also believed to have the power to block such dark influences. As described in chapter 1, this attitude may have reflected an appreciation of the herb's antidepressant effects.

Although the demonic theory of depression passed away long ago, its influence lingers in at least one respect: prejudice toward those who are unlucky enough to suffer from severe depression. Another hangover of the old association between emotional illness and evil was the punitive nature of medical treatments for depression—such as in-discriminate shock treatment—that persisted until a scant three decades ago.

Another software approach to depression grew out of classical Christian theology. This is the idea that sin can eat away at a person's soul if it remains locked up and kept secret. The traditional cure for this interior illness was con-fession, a potentially marvelous religious practice whose healing power is indisputable.

From the confession box, it was only a small step to the client-therapist relationship. Psychotherapy can be seen as a form of confession, in which emotional conflicts un-known even to the patient are brought into the light. But where Christianity focused primarily on sin, psychotherapy devotes its main attention to childhood traumas.

The insights of psychology have taught us the terrible lingering effects of sexual, physical, and emotional abuse suffered during childhood. Treatment for these problems include individual psychotherapy, group therapy, and self-help practices such as "nurturing the inner child."

However, childhood traumas are not the only psycho-logical cause of depression. Social psychology has demon-strated that poverty, lack of social support, and external stressors such as divorce can cause depression. Cognitive psychology has investigated the relationship between de-pression's negative self-talk ("I'm no good") and invented treatments that emphasize deliberate positive internal dia-logue. For example, a client might be encouraged to say "I'm a good person who deserves love and success."

These and other psychological viewpoints have been tremendously influential and until recently were the domi-nant paradigm for analyzing depression. But in recent years the pendulum has swung again. The physical side of depression is once more center stage.

The Rise of the Amine Hypothesis

The new hardware approach to depression is officially called the amine hypothesis. Since its proposal a few decades ago, it has revolutionized attitudes toward depression.

The amine hypothesis states that depression is caused by low levels of certain brain chemicals, called amines because of their chemical similarity to ammonia. Some of the most famous of these amines are serotonin, norepinephrine, and dopamine. According to the amine hypothesis, depression is the result of low levels of these amines.

It was Prozac that brought this theory into public awareness, but the story really goes back to the 1950s and the drug iproniazid. Iproniazid was initially developed for tuberculosis. However, in 1957 scientists discovered that the drug incidentally cured major depression as well. In fact, iproniazid was such an effective antidepressant that within a year it was prescribed to 400,000 patients. It was the first drug of a class later known as the MAO inhibitors.

At the time of this accidental discovery, scientists were already aware that certain amines had the power to influence blood pressure, heart rate, and wakefulness. They knew that the body manufactures these chemicals for its own purposes and then destroys them or reabsorbs them when they've done their job.

When the antidepressant effects of iproniazid were discovered, scientists began to examine its chemical effects in the brain. This investigation soon revealed that iproniazid raises the levels of these biologically active amines, although in an indirect way. It inhibits the enzyme monoamine-oxidase (hence the name monoamine-oxidase inhibitor, or MAO inhibitor for short). The job of monoamine-oxidase is to break down spare amines. When monoamine-oxidase is inhibited by iproniazid, these amines start to build up in higher concentrations.

This bit of information seemed to suggest that depression might actually be caused by a shortage of amines. The idea made sense because some of these amines were known to be used by the nervous system to transmit its signals. Scientists reasoned that a slowdown of the nervous system caused by low amine levels might tend to depress the brain's functions and cause the symptoms of depression. By artificially raising the levels of neurotransmitters, iproniazid would thereby overcome these symptoms.

This altogether sensible idea was given further impetus with the discovery of a new antidepressant, imipramine. Imipramine doesn't inhibit MAO. Scientists investigating its effects were delighted to discover, however, that imipramine has its own way of raising amine levels. Ordinarily, nerve endings send amines across the small distance of a synapse and then reabsorb those amines once the message has been received. This is another method the body uses to prevent amines from building up to excessive levels. But imipramine blocks this reabsorption, the net result being a rise in the levels of norepinephrine and serotonin, and an improvement in depression. The pattern seemed compelling.

A further observation clinched the hypothesis. The blood pressure–lowering drug reserpine was already known to make some people become depressed. Medical investigators were very excited when they discovered that reserpine decreases the level of amines in the brain. Again, low amine levels equals depression. The amine hypothesis was on a roll.

St. John's wort too was scientifically investigated for its influence on brain chemicals. (The results of this research are discussed in chapter 5.) Pharmaceutical companies synthesized new antidepressants that functioned as designer drugs aimed at specific neurotransmitters. More and more people began to take antidepressant medications with good results, and very soon, hardware theories of depression were back on top. Not since the humor theory of medicine had depression been considered a disease of the body itself.

One significant benefit of this revived focus on the physical was to diminish the stigma of depression. Since the Middle Ages, depressed people had had to contend with the additional insult of being considered lazy, crazy, or possessed. With the advent of the amine hypothesis, however, depression could be conceptualized as a "real" illness, a chemical deficiency like diabetes or hypothyroidism.

Depression clearly is a real illness, and brain chemicals are indisputably involved. Nonetheless, the amine hypothesis has some serious problems too.

Flaws in the Amine Hypothesis

Despite the impressive evidence behind it and the drugs it has inspired, the amine hypothesis is clearly not quite right. For one thing, antidepressant drugs raise the levels of biological amines in a few days, at most, and yet the antidepressant effects of these drugs take weeks to emerge. What is going on during this time lag?

Another problem is that different antidepressants, while affecting different amines, work much the same. Some drugs raise serotonin levels; others impact norepinephrine. These are very different chemicals, and it's difficult to accept that they could be interchangeable; but they seem to be. To make matters even more confusing, the drug buproprion (Wellbutrin) does not affect norepinephrine and serotonin levels but still works as well as Prozac—some might even say better.

Obviously, part of the picture is missing; perhaps most of the picture. Upon reflection, this shouldn't be too surprising. There are thousands of active chemicals in the brain. Maybe antidepressants produce their effect by indirectly influencing the levels of as-yet-unidentified chemicals; altering the soup, so to speak, in ways we don't yet understand. Some researchers suspect a role for endorphins and many other specific hormones. However, this all remains speculation.

Unrecognized chemicals aren't the only complication. Scientists have recently discovered that the brain possesses many different kinds of receptors for serotonin and norepinephrine. Antidepressants seem to alter some of these receptors more than others, thereby producing different effects in different parts of the brain. It may be the changed *distribution* of brain chemicals and not their *quantity* that matters most in depression. But this, too, is only a theory.

It will undoubtedly be a long, long time before brain chemistry is fully understood. In the meantime, the truth is that we really don't know how antidepressants work, whether they are drugs or herbs.

And we shouldn't turn our back on software theories, either.

The Big Picture

Realistically, depression is the result of a combination of influences. Traumatic childhood, biological amines, repressed memories, unrecognized brain chemicals, negative self-talk, and special amine receptor sites; all are probably important and mutually influencing. Prozac can facilitate psychotherapy, and psychotherapy can probably raise serotonin levels. The body is all of a piece.

To illustrate the interdependence of causes in depression, I like to use the following analogy. Imagine a car driving on a road littered with nails. The car will probably move rather slowly as the driver tries to steer around the nails. If there are enough nails, however, one will finally puncture a tire, and the car will come to a stop.

In this analogy, it is clearly the nails on the road that are causing the problem. Nonetheless, two cars going down the same road will experience different results. It depends to a great extent on the ruggedness of their tires. Weak tires may suffer a puncture even if there are only a few dull, short nails on the road. But strong tires built with thick layers of rubber and steel can survive all but the biggest, nastiest spikes.

Thus, both internal and external factors matter. And if a car should break down in the middle of such a road, two different kinds of "treatments" would apply. The tires would have to be repaired, but the nails should be removed from the road, as well. Taking care of only one side of this equation will produce temporary relief, at best. The cause of the problem is in the car and on the road; both must be treated for good results.

This story is an allegory to depression. If you grew up in a dysfunctional household, you spent most of your early life "driving carefully" to avoid the spikes of abuse. In order to survive, you had to expend a lot of extra energy, and it inhibited you from living a fully normal life.

Eventually, however, you were injured to some extent. Abusive and shaming words, perhaps even physical and sexual abuse came your way, and you suffered from it. But how much you suffered depended to a great extent on how you were constituted physically. Like the cars in the story, some people are more susceptible to emotional injury than others.

We have all met people who grew up in horrible environments but turned out pretty well, and others who came from decent homes but developed serious emotional problems anyway. This is because of the "tire" side of the question. People are gifted with widely varying genetic backgrounds. Some sets of genes provide tremendous resiliency. Others make a person susceptible to developing depression under the slightest provocation.

Of course, the body is far more complex and sophisticated than an automobile. Unlike a machine, the body has the potential to heal itself. With successful psychotherapy, or even sheer personal determination, the brain may adjust its own brain chemicals and eliminate the symptoms of depression. However, it isn't easy, and if genetic influences toward depression are too strong, it simply can't be done.

It is here that St. John's wort and other antidepressants can be useful. By improving the balance of brain chemicals, antidepressants work on the "tire" side of the equation. With increased energy and elevated mood, everything will become easier. You may gain greater success in psychotherapy and an enhanced ability to make positive life changes.

Maybe you will be able to start exercising more, getting out more, eating better, taking on hobbies you enjoy, and developing better relationships. Once on an upward path there is a win-win cycle, and St. John's wort can help initiate it.

Of course, conventional treatment for depression doesn't include St. John's wort. Drugs are standard care. To see why St. John's wort could be a preferable option, the risks and benefits of pharmaceutical antidepressants must be explored.

CHAPTER FOUR

Conventional Treatment for Depression and Its Drawbacks

- Prozac: Discrepancies between observed side effects and official statistics
- Zoloft and Paxil
- Trazadone and Serzone
- Wellbutrin
- Effexor
- Tricyclics
- MAO inhibitors
- Beyond drugs

Antidepressant drugs have provided enormous benefits to millions of depressed people. However, they can all cause a great variety of side effects, some quite severe. In this chapter I describe some of the benefits and risks of these powerful drugs.

The story of antidepressant drugs begins with iproniazid, the antituberculosis drug found quite by accident to improve depression. Iproniazid was taken off the market after reports circulated that it could cause jaundice. However, in its short tenure it had been so remarkably effective that a search for replacements began in earnest. This effort soon led to two large classes of antidepressants that were to dominate the field for decades: the MAO inhibitors, which work like iproniazid, and the tricyclics, of which imipramine was the first representative.

These early drugs were effective antidepressants but they proved to cause numerous side effects and toxicities. In an attempt to minimize such problems, researchers looked for ways to make the drugs' actions more specific.

MAO inhibitors and, to a lesser extent, the tricyclic drugs are medical shotguns, raising the level of many amines at the same time. Scientists reasoned that perhaps only one of the amines mattered with respect to depression and that the changing levels of other amines were responsible for antidepressant dangers and side effects. By seeking to develop drugs that would work on only one chemical at a time, they hoped they might be able to create a clean medication that would relieve depression and do nothing else.

This was the origin of the selective serotonin-reuptake inhibitors, or SSRIs. This class of drugs, of which Prozac is the most famous representative, specifically raises serotonin levels without affecting other major amines. During their development, the SSRIs proved to be potent antidepressants and far less dangerous when taken in overdose than their predecessors. To the researchers' disappointment, however, the Holy Grail of zero side effects was not achieved. Thus, the search for side-effect-free antidepressants continues.

St. John's wort may in fact fulfill that dream of an anti-depressant with no down side (at least for mild to moderate depression). The herb's benefits are evaluated in chapter 5. First, I will sort through the bewildering array of pharma-ceutical antidepressant options and discuss their strengths and weaknesses. I will also analyze several general problems that confound studies of the safety and efficacy of drugs used for depression.

Prozac

Prozac was the first of the SSRIs to be developed, closely fol-lowed by Zoloft, Paxil, and Serzone. It was the drug that made antidepressants wildly popular, and it remains the most widely prescribed antidepressant drug in history. Pro-zac's appeal lies in its energizing characteristics.

The members of the tricyclic family of antidepressants are all plagued by side effects that work against their value for treating depression: fatigue and sleepiness. Since a sense of low energy is one of the defining characteristics of de-pression, a drug that lowers energy is sharply limited in its benefits as an antidepressant. For catastrophic, major de-pression such a drug might be thought satisfactory. But for mild-to-moderate-depression medications to cause severe fa-tigue renders them next to useless.

The tricyclic drugs produce so much drowsiness that they make excellent sleeping pills. While taking them, it can be difficult to carry out the activities of daily life; and indeed the labeling warns against driving or operating heavy machinery. The prospect of sleeping through life may appeal to some, but most people suffering from depression would rather engage life more fully and successfully. Hence, the great contribution of Prozac. While matching the antidepressant powers of the tricyclic drugs, it simultaneously produces for many people an enhanced sense of energy and alertness—a combination that made Prozac a stunning overnight success.

After this first drug truly useful for mild to moderate depression was out on the market for a while, however, reports began to come back that revealed unexpectedly severe side effects. It turned out that the strength of this drug was also its weakness. Along with increased energy came frequent reports of insomnia, restlessness, agitation, irritability, anxiety, dry mouth, sweating, and palpitations: symptoms, in other words, of excess stimulation.

These effects are strikingly similar to those produced by the classic stimulant drugs, such as caffeine, cocaine, and amphetamine. For this reason, in his popular book *Talking Back to Prozac,* Peter Breggin suggests that Prozac is not a true antidepressant at all. He thinks it should be classed as a stimulant and regulated as a dangerous, potentially addictive drug. Most people would not agree with this radical perspective, but there is no doubt that the stimulating properties of Prozac frequently become a significant problem.

In those for whom insomnia is a part of depression, the drawbacks of Prozac may be evident from the first dose. Falling asleep typically becomes more difficult, and the familiar symptom of early morning awakening grow increasingly intense. As with use of any stimulant, missed sleep may not seem to matter at first. People who have just started taking Prozac say they feel alert and energetic even though they aren't sleeping well. However, after a while the lack of sleep begins to take its toll. The Prozac-initiated alertness begins to feel artificial, memory and concentration become impaired, and as one patient said to me, "I feel like I'm on some kind of binge."

Physicians typically prefer using other antidepressants for their patients with insomnia; or if they do prescribe Prozac, they may prescribe a second drug for use at night. However, some people with depression sleep too much. If you fall into this category, you may find that the stimulating effects of Prozac are just what you need.

Reduced sleeping isn't the only stimulating side effect of Prozac. It can also cause increased daytime agitation and irritability. Many people report a peculiar internal restlessness that makes them fidget incessantly and want to chew gum. Other symptoms include a general increase in anxiety, along with such symptoms as dry mouth, heart palpitations, and hypervigilance. One of my patients said, "I feel like I've drunk ten cups of coffee when I'm on Prozac." Amphetamine abusers describe much the same experience.

To be fair, I should also note that many people feel nothing but a gentle and subtle increase in energy when they take Prozac, and a few even report drowsiness. Many who do experience side effects find that the most unpleasant ones may fade away over time. However, this gradual mellowing does not necessarily occur, and many patients ultimately find Prozac's overstimulation a reason to quit taking it. This unpredictability of results is a phenomenon seen with all drugs and makes a certain amount of individual trial and error unavoidable.

St. John's wort may be a very useful alternative for those who feel hyper on Prozac. Although it, too, is energizing, its effects seem always to be gentle and well tolerated. Excessive stimulation is not the only major problem with Prozac. Many women who use it for several weeks or months complain of a frustrating and usually intolerable side effect, anorgasmia: the inability to experience orgasm. Although sexual arousal may still be possible, orgasm can't be achieved, and these women are left frustrated and unsatisfied.

The official list of Prozac side effects reports anorgasmia as rare, but in clinical practice it is one of the most common reasons patients quit taking the drug. In fact, anorgasmia is so prevalent that at least two competing antidepressants are specifically marketed for not interfering with orgasm (Serzone and Wellbutrin, described later in this chapter). Possible reasons for this discrepancy will be addressed in a separate section devoted to such variances.

In men, this side effect can manifest as difficulty achieving ejaculation or frank impotence, but such problems are less frequent than female anorgasmia. Some men even appreciate this side effect. They find that Prozac successfully treats premature ejaculation and may take it specifically for that purpose.

Besides interfering with orgasm, Prozac can also cause a decrease in libido. This side effect occurs in both men and women, and it can be extremely unpleasant. One patient said to me, "I like feeling less depressed but sex just doesn't seem to exist for me anymore. It's like a part of me has been chopped out."

Another common side effect of Prozac is headache. Indeed, according to the official statistics, 20 percent of patients on Prozac develop headaches. This is not quite as problematic as it sounds, however, because 15 percent of the patients given placebo in the official studies also developed headaches. The mere thought of taking a drug, it appears, is enough to make one's head hurt.

Nevertheless, the headaches caused by Prozac can be severe, probably more severe than placebo headaches. Several patients of mine developed full-blown migraine attacks for the first time in their lives when they started Prozac, and in a few cases it took a month or two afterwards to resolve this problem. However, it is yet another example of the unpredictability of drugs that Prozac actually *prevents* migraines in some people.

Other physical problems caused by Prozac include nausea and diarrhea. According to official statistics, 21.1 percent of those who take Prozac develop nausea and 12.3 percent develop diarrhea, and these numbers appear to coincide fairly well with clinical experience. Weight loss due to loss of appetite may also occur, although seldom dramatically enough to make Prozac an effective diet pill.

Another common complaint of people who take Prozac is that they "can't think straight." I have mentioned how drug-induced sleep deprivation can cause impaired memory and concentration, but Prozac seems to cause these side effects directly in some patients. Symptoms include walking into a room and not remembering why, forgetting appointments, and being unable to stay on a single train of thought.

The most dramatic adverse effects attributed to Prozac concern the specter of increased violence toward self or others. This charge first appeared in 1990, when Dr. Martin Teicher of McLean Hospital reported that six of his depressed patients had suddenly developed intense suicidal tendencies upon starting Prozac. Subsequently, several lawsuits were instituted claiming that Prozac had caused violent criminal aggression. Overnight Prozac gained the reputation of being a killer drug.

It is easy to be misled, however, by anecdotal reports. Most of the violent acts attributed to Prozac use were committed by people with a previous history of violence. Did Prozac cause that violence, or was it just a convenient excuse? And suicide is a classic feature of depression itself. Could it be that what seemed to be a suicide brought on by Prozac was only a suicide Prozac failed to prevent? Since more people were taking Prozac than had ever taken any other antidepressant before, the number of individual cases of suicide while on Prozac would naturally be comparatively higher.

Indeed, careful evaluation of the data showed that on a percentage basis people taking Prozac didn't commit suicide any more often than those taking the older antidepressants. This mathematical analysis soothed substantially the public's fears and restored confidence. Whatever else might be said about it, Prozac is not a murderer.

This piece of information isn't the last word on the subject, however. On *average*, Prozac probably *reduces* the suicide rate in depressed people, by treating their depression. It is still possible, nonetheless, that Prozac may increase the potential for suicide in *certain* individuals. That is certainly Martin Teicher's impression, and there is no reason to dispute his words. Drugs can cause in a few individuals effects that don't occur in the majority of people who take them. Prozac may present a real danger of violence to a small subset of the population.

A potentially more serious unresolved concern regarding the posafety of Prozac is the possibility of long-term side effects. It is far more difficult to establish the safety of a drug over an extended period than to determine immediate adverse consequences. Safety tests for drugs are very seldom carried beyond eight weeks. If Prozac were to cause side effects after, say, fifteen years of use, there is no way to know now; the drug simply hasn't been in use that long.

Actually, long-term risks are not known for most drugs. These are typically discovered only by accident; and if they occur rarely, they would be very difficult to identify. But most drugs are taken to prevent relatively serious medical complications. For example, with high blood pressure–lowering drugs intended to prevent heart attacks and strokes, a small risk of unknown harm would be worth taking for their dramatic benefit.

Similarly, major depression is a disease that can cause death. Using antidepressants to prevent immediate harm may be worth the risk of unknown consequences. Life involves trade-offs. But Prozac is now being used almost casually. Doctors are prescribing it for a great variety of symptoms—from PMS to premature ejaculation—and the implicit trade-off of short-term benefit versus long-term risk may not be worth it for many of these conditions.

The biggest concern is that Prozac may cause a delayed syndrome that falls within the family of tardive dyskinesia. This is a disease caused by prolonged use of drugs that treat schizophrenia. A syndrome of abnormal movements (dyskinesias), as its name implies, can develop after years, or even decades, of taking antischizophrenic medication (thus they are "tardy" symptoms). The uncontrollable movements of tardive dyskinesia are quite unpleasant, involving lip smacking, tongue rolling, and facial grimacing.

The worst part of this syndrome is that it doesn't necessarily go away on discontinuing medication. Tardive dyskinesia is often forever.

There is no guarantee that Prozac won't produce its own syndrome in people who take it for a long time; and there's considerable reason to suspect it might. Although tardive dyskinesia isn't understood completely, it seems to be a kind of permanent version of typical antischizophrenic side effects. What if the excessively energizing effects of Prozac could become permanent, too, leading to a syndrome of unrelenting agitation, restlessness, and insomnia? Purely speculation at this point; but considering the history of disastrous side effects caused by other drugs, perhaps it should be taken seriously.

Whatever its long-term implications, Prozac has shown low immediate toxicity. Patients who have attempted to commit suicide with Prozac have generally experienced only relatively mild symptoms from overdose, such as vomiting and agitation, although seizures have also occurred in rare instances.

Why Does the Official List of Prozac's Side Effects Look So Good?

Despite the problems previously described, the official statistics on Prozac's side effects show a drug that seems to be almost side-effect-free. The *Physicians' Desk Reference (PDR)* lists an incidence of sexual side effects, for example, that is under 2 percent. This seems to be so different from the clinical experience of practitioners that there has to be an explanation. And there is.

At first glance, Prozac's manufacturer, Eli Lilly, did a very careful job of screening for side effects. The *PDR* states that side-effect frequencies were determined from a pool of 1,730 patients involved in placebo-controlled clinical trials. This sounds impressive, but a close analysis shows many potential sources for error.

Perhaps the most obvious problem is that these studies lasted for only four to six weeks. Anorgasmia often takes somewhat longer than that to develop, and even if it did occur in that interval, women might not immediately connect the symptom with the drug. Thus, to detect anorgasmia the screening period was simply too short.

This limitation is compounded by the fact that a great many people dropped out of the Prozac studies early. According to Peter Breggin in *Talking Back to Prozac,* only 286 patients actually completed the four- to six-week trials used as the basis for FDA approval. This is a very small number indeed, not nearly enough on which to base firm conclusions about side-effect frequencies.

But there is yet another reason not to rely on the official side-effects reports. Good interviewing technique is essential for reliable results, especially with regard to sensitive subjects, such as sexual dysfunction. Many patients may simply not be willing to admit such problems. Studies performed by researchers experienced in the field of sexual dysfunction have shown substantially higher rates of such problems in people taking antidepressants, perhaps as high as 1 in 3.[1]

In clinical experience, practically all of the major Prozac side effects seem to occur far more often than officially recognized. The official side-effects percentages are probably far off the mark.

How Well Does Prozac Actually Work for Depression?

The answer to this fundamental question remains unclear, not only for Prozac but for all antidepressants. Depression is not easy to evaluate scientifically. Unlike high blood pressure or diabetes, the extent of a person's depression can't be measured by a machine. Depression is primarily a subjective experience, and there is no way to get around depending on the patient's own reports and the physician's personal impression. Difficult to duplicate and susceptible to the influence of suggestion, these reports and impressions are highly variable.

In order to achieve some sort of objectivity, experimenters use a special interview technique called the Hamilton Depression Rating Scale (HAM-D). Administered by a physician, the HAM-D is a test that takes into account physical signs, such as slowed speech and movement, as well as answers to questions, such as "Do you frequently cry for no reason?" and "Do you feel fatigued?" Each observation and answer is turned into a number, and a total HAM-D score is created by combining all these numbers. Higher numbers indicate greater depression.

The HAM-D interview and others like it are widely used in studies evaluating the effectiveness of antidepressant drugs. In a typical clinical trial, some patients are given placebo, and others real drug. The HAM-D test is then administered at intervals, and the resulting numbers are compared to evaluate effects on depression of drug and placebo.

Unfortunately, while the HAM-D is much more reliable than simply asking doctors to decide whether patients seem to improve or not, the scale still leaves a lot to be desired. One difficulty is that different scores may result when various physicians administer the HAM-D to the same patient. For best results, it is recommended that all the physicians involved in a study learn the use of the HAM-D from a single teacher in order to make their rating styles similar. But this step is often skipped, and even when it is followed, the results remain far from consistent. Different doctors' assessments may still differ widely, and, as shown in the following text, there is plenty of room for the influence of suggestion.

Limitations in the reliability of HAM-D aren't the only obstacles to obtaining reliable estimates of Prozac's effectiveness. A potentially more serious problem lies in the nature of controlled experiments themselves.

In a proper double-blind study, neither the doctor nor the patient can tell the difference between placebo and drug. In other words, they are both "blind" in order to prevent the power of suggestion from skewing the results.

When people know they are taking a real drug, they have a strong inclination to expect results, which may actually produce them. The reverse naturally occurs for placebo. Similarly, a doctor aware of what is in a capsule may inadvertently communicate positive or negative suggestion by body language or tone of voice. To keep a test unbiased, it is essential that there is no way to tell placebo and real medication apart. They are usually packaged identically, and their identity is kept secret from all but a committee overseeing the experiment.

Since Prozac causes so many side effects, however, patients taking Prozac may be perfectly aware that what they are getting isn't placebo. The difference may be as immediately apparent to them as that between coffee and decaf.

Thus, a seemingly double-blind experiment could in fact be perfectly transparent.

This loss of blinding means that the power of suggestion can creep in, and the power of suggestion should never be underestimated. Years of experience have shown that positive expectation has the power to improve almost all diseases. Considering all the media hype surrounding Prozac, its suggestive power may be very great indeed.

Patients who believe they are taking an effective drug are inclined to take an optimistic view of their symptoms and typically persuade themselves they are feeling better. This can lead to improved HAM-D scores. But a placebo can do more than that; it can actually speed up recovery. This is known to be the case for many illnesses, including such objective ones as infections; and when the disease is already a psychological one, psychological influences are undoubtedly even stronger. Depressed patients who know they are being given Prozac may say to themselves, "Since I'm taking a powerful drug, I'm going to be less depressed soon." This will create a kind of positive self-talk that can be as beneficial as expensive psychotherapy.

Furthermore, Prozac's particular side effects may enhance the drug's placebo potential because these effects relate specifically to the disease being treated. Stimulant effects simulate relief from depression, which may convince patients that their depression is lifting, providing their imaginations with more fodder for positive thinking. There's nothing wrong with positive suggestion, of course. However, it can obscure determining the effectiveness of Prozac per se.

Physicians have implicit faith in the power of drugs, too—especially new drugs. This faith might distort the outcome of Prozac-placebo comparison experiments in the following manner: By observing increased fidgeting or from the patient's reports of increased insomnia, a doctor administering the HAM-D may come to suspect that a particular patient is taking Prozac rather than a placebo. This suspicion may be conscious or unconscious. In either case, when administering the HAM-D, the doctor may inadvertently skew his or her observations to reflect expectation of improvement.

Thus, the effects of suggestion may be influencing trials of Prozac (and other antidepressants) in numerous unforeseen ways. This problem might be overcome by using caffeine as a placebo instead of sugar. However, this has never been tried. We are therefore in the position of not really knowing how much of Prozac's apparent benefit is due to this hidden placebo effect.

There is only one situation in which it doesn't matter very much whether double-blind tests remain blind. That is when the results are so dramatic that the influence of positive suggestion is completely outclassed. For example, when penicillin was first used to treat pneumonia, doctors didn't need double-blind studies to tell them that it worked. The effects in terms of saving lives were immediately obvious.

If Prozac were as powerful for depression as penicillin is for pneumonia, we could dispense with all this caviling about double-blind experiments. Unfortunately, Prozac isn't that dramatically effective. It often fails—far more often than penicillin fails to cure pneumonia. Peter Breggin reports that in quite a few of the initial Prozac studies, the drug didn't surpass placebo at all. Other research showed it less effective than the older drug imipramine. And a surprising number of the studies that did show favorable results had to juggle the statistics considerably to produce an apparent benefit. Some used questionable procedures, such as deliberately leaving out reports on some of the patients or comparing Prozac's results at six weeks with placebo results at two weeks.

In the absence of overwhelming evidence for Prozac's effectiveness, we must take the influence of suggestion seriously. Thus, we cannot fully rely on any of the studies performed and have to conclude that the precise rate of effectiveness of Prozac remains unknown. This surprising flaw in the research record applies to all other antidepressants as well.

Zoloft and Paxil

These two drugs are copycats of Prozac produced by competing drug companies. The term *copycat* isn't quite fair because, while these medications function somewhat similarly to Prozac, they are chemically distinct and sometimes produce different clinical effects. Occasionally, when one member of the Prozac-Zoloft-Paxil group fails, another succeeds.

On average, none of the drugs in this triad has been shown to be better than another with regard to efficacy or the extent of side effects. But some *individuals* do better with one than another. The situation is similar to what is commonly seen in results from the many anti-inflammatory pills used for pain. Overall, they are pretty similar, but certain people respond best to a particular drug from among that family of drugs.

A dramatic example of this phenomenon occurred one day in my private practice: Two patients who didn't know each other came in one right after the other. They both were complaining of pain from a sprained ankle. The first one told me she had tried Naprosyn without luck, but when she switched to ibuprofen, she felt immediately better. The other patient told me exactly the reverse of that story. Individual variation of this type is completely normal; and the advantage to having a variety of drugs to choose from is that if one causes too many side effects, there is a list of options.

Generally, Paxil tends to be the least stimulating of the three drugs. It actually causes tiredness in a significant number of patients who take it. This may make it preferable for patients who suffer from anxiety and insomnia, and less useful for those who complain of fatigue and excessive sleep. Zoloft stands somewhere in the middle, while Prozac is the most energizing. But these are only average effects, and there are wide individual variations.

Frequency of headaches, nausea, and confusion seems to be roughly similar among users of these drugs. However, patients may develop certain side effects in response to one drug and not another. Nonetheless, when sexual side effects occur from one of these drugs for a particular patient, they will often occur with all of them.

Trazadone and Serzone

Trazadone is one of the first serotonin-specific drugs developed, although it isn't an SSRI and doesn't raise serotonin levels as dramatically as Prozac. The biggest problem with trazadone is that it causes tremendous drowsiness. Because of this overwhelming side effect, trazadone has come to be used more widely as a sleeping pill than as an antidepressant. It is one of the drugs commonly given in combination with stimulating antidepressants to counteract drug-induced insomnia.

Serzone is known unofficially as "son of trazadone," and it usually isn't classified as an SSRI either. Its particular claim to fame is that unlike other SSRIs it doesn't seem to cause a high incidence of sexual dysfunction. In advertising, the manufacturer trumpets this characteristic, offering Serzone as a less side-effect-ridden replacement for Prozac.

Serzone has thus far failed, however, to make a major impact. It causes less drowsiness than trazadone, but its effect still tends toward somnolence. As one patient described it, "When I'm on Serzone I feel like I'm swimming through soup." Serzone is useful primarily for patients in whom anxiety and insomnia are a significant component of depression.

Wellbutrin

This drug narrowly missed *being* Prozac. It was approved as an antidepressant in 1985, two years before Prozac's release; and if it weren't for early reports of increased seizure activity in patients using it, Peter Kramer's book would probably have been called *Listening to Wellbutrin.*

The high incidence of seizures reported during premarketing trials of Wellbutrin held it back. Although it was eventually discovered that Wellbutrin could be safe when used correctly, its reputation was tainted and its release delayed. Prozac was already firmly established as the dominant antidepressant by the time Wellbutrin came back into circulation.

Many physicians remain leery of prescribing Wellbutrin out of fear of causing seizures. If too high a dose is taken at one time, or if Wellbutrin is combined with certain other drugs, the risk of seizure can reach almost 4 percent. Nonetheless, Wellbutrin is a useful medication when used carefully. Its great advantage is that, although it is fully as energizing as Prozac, it doesn't cause sexual dysfunction. Like Prozac, Wellbutrin can cause insomnia, agitation, restlessness, and anxiety, as well as nausea, headache, and dry mouth.

The mechanism of action in Wellbutrin remains completely unknown. It produces no significant effect on norepinephrine or serotonin and only weakly increases levels of the biological amine dopamine, thus confounding the amine hypothesis of depression. Wellbutrin proves that we don't understand the biological basis of depression.

Effexor

Although Prozac's original claim to fame was that its action was specific, with Effexor we come full circle. Its manufacturer seems particularly proud of the fact that it raises both norepinephrine and serotonin levels. Unlike older antidepressants that do the same thing, however, Effexor usually produces an energizing effect.

Effexor is frequently tried when SSRIs fail. It typically produces a higher incidence of some side effects than the Prozac-Paxil-Zoloft triad, particularly nausea, but it doesn't seem to impair orgasm as often as the SSRIs. Otherwise, the side effects are rather similar.

Tricyclics

Prior to the release of Prozac, the most widely used family of drugs belonged to a category known as tricyclic antidepressants. This name comes from the three circular chemical structures found in the tricyclic molecule. Imipramine was the first tricyclic antidepressant, and subsequent drugs in the family all bear striking similarities. Some of the more famous are Elavil (amitriptyline), Sinequan (doxepin), and Pamelor (nortriptyline).

All of these antidepressants have demonstrable effectiveness in the treatment of major depression. Nevertheless, they cause too many side effects to be useful in the treatment of mild to moderate depression. The tricyclics were originally derived from antihistamines, and they still carry the entire list of classic antihistamine side effects, such as drowsiness, blurred vision, dry mouth, constipation, sweating, heart palpitations, weight gain, dizziness, and urinary retention. Sometimes these side effects can be even greater in the antidepressants than the antihistamines because of the high dosages necessary to produce full antidepressant benefits.

Recently, antihistamines have been developed that are relatively side-effect-free, such as Claritin. But the tricyclic drugs are more similar to the oldest antihistamines, such as Benedryl, which is sold over the counter as a sleeping pill. The tricyclic antidepressants make excellent sleeping pills, too. (And most of them are pretty decent antihistamines, as well!) Other common side effects include fainting, sexual dysfunction, and weight gain (sometimes massive). Tricyclic drugs can also cause seizures and injury to the heart.

With side effects like these, it's hard to tell you're not depressed. Drowsiness, dry mouth, and weight gain may be a reasonable price to pay for relief from major depression. But for mild to moderate depression, the side effects of these older antidepressants are often worse than the disease—and depressing in their own right.

In *Listening to Prozac*, Peter Kramer speculates for many pages on why Prozac took off in a way the tricyclic antidepressants never did. He wonders whether Prozac "touches features of depression" Pamelor can't reach and hypothesizes that serotonin may be more fundamentally related to depression than the amines raised by tricyclics (primarily norepinephrine). But there is a simpler explanation that is more likely: side effects.

Pamelor causes more side effects than Prozac, and the ones it causes are precisely the ones you don't want if you suffer from mild to moderate depression. Prozac's immediate stimulation creates a positive suggestion of recovery from depression, while Pamelor's drowsiness connotes deepening illness. Thus, both the side effects of tricyclics and the suggestions that they provide to the imagination are exactly wrong. Tricyclics simply aren't good drugs for treatment of mild to moderate depression.

MAO Inhibitors

This is the oldest category of antidepressants, and if it weren't for the known risks they pose, the MAO inhibitors would be much more widely used. Representative drugs include Marplan (isocarboxazid), Nardil (Phenylzine), and Parnate (tranylcypromine).

Drugs in this family inhibit the enzyme monoamine-oxidase, a "garbage cleaner" enzyme in charge of breaking down excess biological amines. When monoamine-oxidase is poisoned, the levels of numerous brain chemicals begin to rise. The MAO inhibitors are some of the most powerful antidepressants known, perhaps because of their wide spectrum of action. They are energizing and can produce dramatic reductions in symptoms. Unfortunately, they cause many side effects and can even cause death if not used with extreme care.

The dangers of these drugs come directly from the way they work. The job of the MAO-scavenger enzyme is to control the levels of biological amines. When a person takes an MAO inhibitor, the amine levels naturally begin to rise. The goal is to raise them just enough to help combat depression. However, there's a fine line between just enough and too much. If the levels of biological amines pass a certain threshold, they begin to cause extremely high blood pressure and the risk of death by brain hemorrhage.

The usual cause of this catastrophe is additional amines taken by mouth. Numerous other drugs contain amines, such as Ritalin, ephedrine, pseudoephedrine (Sudafed), phenylpropanolamine (also found in over-the-counter cold and allergy remedies), and asthma medications. A person on MAO inhibitors must avoid these medications religiously. (Prozac, tricyclic antidepressants, insulin, oral diabetes drugs, and antabuse can also cause serious reactions in someone taking an MAO inhibitor, but by other mechanisms.)

Drugs aren't the only problem. The MAO inhibitors are among the few medications where watching what you eat is required, as well. A substance called tyramine occurs in many foods, and it is a natural relative of the body's biologically active amines. If a tyramine-containing food is consumed by a patient taking an MAO inhibitor, this may be enough to trigger a fatal reaction. Dangerous foods include cheese, dried meat, dried fish, canned figs, broad beans, and concentrated yeast products, as well as vermouth and other wines. Patients taking MAO inhibitors must treat these common foods as deadly poisons.

Because of this unique risk and the dietary challenge it presents, MAO inhibitors are only rarely used today. However, they are still tried sometimes when all else fails.

Beyond Drugs

Although drug therapy is rapidly becoming the mainstay of conventional treatment for depression, it isn't the only accepted approach. Conventional medicine still accepts the benefit of psychotherapy, although sometimes grudgingly, because treatment of psychological disorders simply doesn't fit the medical model very well. Doctors are much more comfortable prescribing drugs.

One problem plaguing psychotherapy's acceptance is that its effectiveness is next to impossible to evaluate scientifically. Double-blind experiments are difficult even to conceive. Nonetheless, what research has been performed seems to indicate that psychotherapy can be an effective treatment for depression.

One great advantage of psychotherapy is that, unlike drugs, it can produce positive effects that "belong to you." These benefits continue long after therapy stops and may enrich the rest of your life. But psychotherapy is expensive, time consuming, and not always successful. Should psychotherapy not work fully, or if it simply isn't an option, taking an antidepressant drug may prove useful. And yet, considering all the side effects of drugs, St. John's wort might be an even better choice for mild to moderate depression. From the chapter that follows, you will learn how to treat depression with this safe, natural, and essentially side-effect-free herb.

CHAPTER FIVE

St. John's Wort: A Safe and Effective Alternative Treatment for Depression

- A story
- What research says about St. John's wort's effectiveness
- Theories about how it works
- What clinicians who prescribe it say
- Side effects

Alternative medicine includes many unproved and worthless treatments. However, St. John's wort does not fall into either of these categories. Both its effectiveness and its side effects have been evaluated in studies fully as large, long, and rigorous as those used to validate Prozac and other prescription drugs. Much of that evidence is presented in this chapter. But first I'd like to illustrate how significant St. John's wort's effects can be.

A Story

Laura was a forty-three-year-old mother of three who had been plagued with depression her whole life. The cause was undoubtedly the shaming and verbal abuse that she experienced throughout her upbringing; but even after years of effective psychotherapy, her symptoms of depression lingered like a habit she couldn't break. Laura felt chronically blue, empty, and fatigued. Although she was never suicidal, she felt that she wasn't really living. The stresses of life left Laura so drained that by eight o'clock every night she didn't have enough energy left for anything but brushing her teeth and going to bed. Most weekends she spent lying on the couch whenever possible. "I'm coping and that's all I'm doing," she would say.

Laura's husband had been sympathetic, but he began spending more and more time apart from her. He wanted to take walks in the evening, play golf on the weekends, and go traveling from time to time. Although he would have preferred to do all these things with his wife, she was always too tired. He felt he needed to enjoy himself even if Laura couldn't join in. So he started to spend more time with his friends.

Laura felt that she and her husband were drifting apart. Her first response was to start going to sleep even earlier. Then something inside her woke up and told her she'd better do something positive before it was too late.

Laura's family doctor had been urging her for two years to try Prozac. Her particular kind of depression, with its chronic fatigue and excessive sleeping, seemed to make her a perfect candidate for this antidepressant. Laura had always demurred on the grounds that she didn't believe in taking drugs. However, now she felt ready to try anything. With a sigh of satisfaction, the doctor prescribed a single 20 milligram dose of Prozac daily.

Unfortunately, things didn't go well. From the very first dose, Laura experienced unpleasant side effects. Her sleep, never restful, became broken and racked by nightmares. During the day she felt uneasy and on edge. She would startle violently when her husband entered the room unexpectedly or her seven-year-old screeched in play, and her heart would start racing and palpitating.

However, Laura did feel more energetic, and she began to get out with her husband more often. They took a trip to visit relatives in Minnesota, and once or twice they played golf on the weekends. For a little while she felt optimistic that their intimacy was returning, until the gradual development of sexual side effects rose up as a new obstacle. First orgasm became difficult, then impossible, and finally all desire disappeared. As Laura described the experience, "You'd think my body was made of wood the way it reacts. I don't feel anything. Sex is only a memory."

Sympathetic to her situation, Laura's doctor tried a succession of alternative medications. The results, unfortunately, were less than impressive. Paxil gave her headaches and made her more fatigued than ever, Zoloft caused exactly the same side effects as Prozac, Effexor made Laura "want to throw up night and day," and Serzone put her "into a trance so deep I didn't know if I was there or somewhere else."

And each time she stopped taking a drug, Laura sank back into her usual depression and the intolerable habits from constant fatigue. She felt trapped. She couldn't accept either her old depression or the side effects the drugs caused. It was in this state of frustration that she finally came to me.

"I don't know if there's anything that can help me without poisoning me," she said, "but if there is I want to try it."

I started Laura on a standard dose of St. John's wort, for which details follow, and asked her to come back once a week to tell me how she was doing. Strictly speaking, such frequent appointments aren't necessary, but I suspected she might, without encouragement, give up on the herb. I knew she was used to experiencing side effects, and I reasoned that she might misinterpret the gentleness of St. John's wort as ineffectiveness.

This fear was proved justified when she came back for her first follow-up. "It's not doing anything," she said. "I'm back to my same old drudge of a self." When I asked her about side effects she said, "Nothing, not a thing. I don't think there's anything in those capsules."

I encouraged her to be patient. "You wanted a treatment that didn't cause side effects," I reminded her. "Now that you have it, don't give up before it has time to work. Remember, I said that you might have to wait four to eight weeks."

My reassurance kept her going for another two weeks, but at the beginning of week four, she was ready to throw in the towel. "I think I'm going to have to go back to drugs," she said.

It took all my powers of persuasion to keep her going. "I think I notice a difference in you already," I said, quite sincerely. "You don't look quite so depressed. I think you just can't recognize it because you're so used to getting side effects along with feeling better."

It was something about her eyes that seemed different to me, but it wasn't until week six that Laura could notice the change herself. "It suddenly dawned on me the other day," she said, "that I don't feel so empty." I thought she looked considerably brighter and told her so.

By the eighth week it was obvious that St. John's wort was doing its job. "I feel like a human being when I get up in the morning," Laura said, smiling. "I have enough energy to enjoy myself. I'm not just getting by; I feel like I'm starting to live."

But she was amazed at how gradually it all happened. "I couldn't tell anything at all for the longest time. But looking back I'd say that taking St. John's wort was like filling up a lake drop by drop. Almost without my being aware of it, the emptiness and hopelessness were gradually replaced by a quiet sense of calm."

Laura was impressed by the difference between St. John's wort and drug therapy. "Taking Prozac was like being shot in the face with a firehose," she said. "It worked, but it was violent and unpleasant. And the other drugs were each just as bad in their own ways."

On St. John's wort, Laura found a new ability to manage stress. "I can't believe how calm I feel. It's like I have a reservoir inside, something I can dip into when I need it. Before I was scraping the bottom of the barrel for something I didn't have."

Laura's story is fairly typical of those for whom St. John's wort is successful, and I tell it here to paint a picture of what the herb can do. However, anecdotal evidence doesn't prove anything, and the history of medicine is littered with testimonials to the effectiveness of "cures" that don't really work. To prove a treatment is effective, research is essential. The evidence for St. John's wort is among the strongest in all alternative medicine.

What Research Says About St. John's Wort's Effectiveness

According to a report in the August 1996 edition of the *British Medical Journal,* there have now been twenty-three randomized double-blind clinical trials of St. John's wort in the treatment of depression.[2] The total number of patients involved in these studies has reached a respectable 1,757, presenting a compelling case for this traditional herbal treatment. One to two thousand is a typical total number of participants for drug validation trials.[3] Thus, St. John's wort has earned the right to be taken seriously.

Some of these studies compared St. John's wort against placebo, while others compared St. John's wort against a pharmaceutical antidepressant. This chapter covers comparisons between St. John's wort and placebo, leaving the herb-drug comparisons for chapter 7.

One of the studies that most impresses conventional physicians is a four-week comparison of St. John's wort and placebo performed in 1993 by the German physician K. D.

Hansgen and his colleagues.[4] In this study seventy-two patients from eleven different physicians' practices were selected based on standard *DSM (Diagnostic Statistical Manual of Mental Disorders)* criteria for major depression. The study design followed in every way the research used to validate pharmaceutical antidepressants.

In order to quantify the extent of improvement produced by St. John's wort, Hansgen used the systematic rating scale for depression, the HAM-D test. As you may recall from my earlier explanation, the HAM-D combines physicians' observations and patients' answers to questions to yield a number that represents the severity of depression. Higher numbers indicate more serious depression and lower numbers, milder.

At the beginning of this study, patients were given HAM-D tests to determine the starting levels of their depression. Then, half the participants were given a standard dose of St. John's wort, the other half placebo. At two and four weeks, the patients were retested and their scores recorded.

Patients taking St. John's wort showed remarkable improvement. Their HAM-D scores dropped from an average of 21.8 prior to treatment to 9.2 after four weeks of treatment. This drop of almost 60 percent compares quite favorably to what is usually seen with antidepressant medication.

As always happens (although it never ceases to surprise), patients taking placebo also improved. However, their average HAM-D score only dropped by about 30 percent, from an initial average of 20.4 to 14.7. Statistically, this difference in results was highly significant.

Another way of looking at this data is that 81 percent of the patients taking St. John's wort improved significantly (greater than a 50 percent drop in their scores), while only

26 percent of the placebo group responded. Again, this was a statistically significant result.

Three patients on placebo dropped out of the study because their symptoms of depression became too severe to continue. This did not happen in the St. John's wort group.

The psychiatrists involved in the study also used two other methods of measuring levels of depression to confirm the HAM-D results, and these measurements gave substantially the same result. Overall, the difference in outcomes between patients on placebo and those on St. John's wort easily exceeded the requirements for statistical significance.

During the course of this study, only one patient taking St. John's wort reported any adverse effect (disturbance in sleep), while two patients on placebo said they developed stomach upset.

The scientific quality of this study was as good as any used to prove the effectiveness of a drug treatment for depression. Its method of randomization followed standard guidelines, the techniques of statistical analysis used were mathematically acceptable, study dropouts were accounted for, adverse reactions were indicated, and the double-blind method was preserved throughout.

In one sense at least, this study was superior to typical antidepressant versus placebo trials: that of a true double-blind test. Drugs cause side effects, and as I pointed out in the preceding chapter, those effects may allow patients to distinguish between drug and placebo, even when they look exactly alike. Thus, the influence of the power of suggestion cannot be excluded. This makes the legitimacy of all double-blind studies for traditional antidepressant medication somewhat suspect. No similar problem occurs with the essentially side-effect-free St. John's wort.

While this multicenter study makes a compelling case for St. John's wort, a total of seventy-two patients (minus dropouts) is not enough by itself to establish the effectiveness of a treatment. Therefore, an additional thirty-six patients were added to the trial in 1996, and the study methodology was repeated.[5] The results followed exactly the same pattern as before.

The Hansgen study involved patients whose depression was moderately severe. In a separate study, the effectiveness of St. John's wort was evaluated for mildly depressed patients (with an average HAM-D of about 16). The 105 participants were drawn from three physicians' practices and followed for four weeks.[6] At the end of the study, 67 percent of the patients on St. John's wort showed satisfactory response to treatment (a greater than 50 percent reduction in their HAM-D scores), compared to only 28 percent of those patients on placebo. Significant improvements were particularly noted in mood, anxiety, and insomnia.

One of the longest studies on St. John's wort was performed in 1991. It followed 50 patients for eight weeks, and once more the herb proved significantly more effective than placebo.[7] Yet another multicenter study, performed in 1991, showed positive results in 116 patients followed for six weeks.[8] This study suffered, however, from one significant drawback: The St. John's wort was administered in the form of drops, which may have been distinguishable by taste from placebo.

In 1995 E. Ernst published a formal review of the literature, ranking the trials based on standard scientific criteria and eliminating those with significant flaws.[9] Out of the 1,757 combined total of participants in these randomized double-blind studies of St. John's wort versus placebo, Ernst narrowed the field to 902 patients who were involved in studies of the highest caliber. The cumulative results of these carefully selected trials were impressive. Ernst reported that "taken together, these data are scientifically compelling and leave little doubt as to the efficacy of Hypericum [St. John's wort] in the treatment of depressive symptoms."

Despite this solid research evidence, physicians in the United States and the United Kingdom still find it difficult to accept the legitimacy of an herbal treatment such as St. John's wort. It is almost amusing to watch this bias play out in published editorial comments. The favorable review of St. John's wort published in the August 1996 edition of the *British Medical Journal* triggered a critical response in the same issue.[10,11] Although the physician-authors of this editorial reluctantly acknowledge that the published studies are "promising," they spend the bulk of the article attacking research into St. John's wort as not sufficiently scientific.

"None lasted longer than six weeks," they point out, which is too short a time "to assess the risk of relapse and the possibility of late side effects." The studies "lack diagnostic precision" because some do not classify carefully enough the type of depression under study. And "the observers in these multicentre [*sic*] trials" may not have received special training to ensure identical results on the HAM-D evaluation.

These are all valid points. *However, every one of these criticisms, and more, apply to the research into Prozac, too.* For example, in the 1997 *Physicians' Desk Reference* the manufacturer of Prozac states that "the effectiveness of Prozac in long-term use, that is, for more than 5 to 6 weeks, has not been systematically evaluated in controlled trials."[12] Why should St. John's wort be forced to adhere to a higher standard than that required for drugs?

Whether consciously or unconsciously, criticisms such as those in the *BMJ* article are strongly influenced by physician bias against herbal treatment. Analysis of the causes of this bias is presented in chapter 9. Suffice it to say for now that were St. John's wort a drug there is little doubt it would already be approved for use in both the United Kingdom and the United States.

How Does St. John's Wort Work?

As explained in chapter 4, science doesn't really understand how pharmaceutical antidepressants produce their effects. The prevailing theory is that low levels of biological amines (such as serotonin and norepinephrine) are responsible for depression and that antidepressants function by raising those levels. However, there are many problems with this "amine hypothesis," not the least of which is that some antidepressants function perfectly well without significantly changing the level of any biological amines.

The amine hypothesis must be only part of the story. Nonetheless, it's the only explanation we have thus far. For this reason, researchers have investigated whether St. John's wort changes amine levels, too. The results remain inconclusive.

Early research seemed to indicate that extracts of St. John's wort inhibit the enzyme monoamine-oxidase.[13] This indication placed the herb in the MAO inhibitor class of antidepressants and spawned a series of warnings about not eating certain foods while taking it (see "Warnings" in the next chapter). However these studies involved applying extracts of St. John's wort directly into test tubes. Later investigation showed that the dosages of St. John's wort taken orally in actual practice are probably far too low to inhibit monoamine-oxidase.[14] MAO inhibition is no longer considered a likely explanation for St. John's wort's effectiveness in treating depression.

More recent research suggests that St. John's wort may actually function by inhibiting the reuptake of serotonin. In one study, researchers added St. John's wort to test tubes filled with primeval nerve cells and observed that serotonin receptors seemed to be suppressed.[15] They theorized that the herb might therefore function by impairing the reuptake of serotonin into cells.

This highly theoretical study did not, however, investigate whether normal dosages of St. John's wort can raise serotonin levels. Another study attempted to answer this practical question by examining the brains of rats and mice who were fed St. John's wort extracts.[16] Serotonin and dopamine levels did rise significantly in treated animals. Nevertheless, this experiment produced a surprising finding: A preparation of St. John's wort in which the presumed active ingredient hypericin was removed still caused the same effect.

Thus, the only safe conclusion is that we really do not know how St. John's wort works in treating depression. However, this only puts St. John's wort in the good company of all other antidepressants, whose methods of function remain unclear, as well.

What Clinicians Who Prescribe It Say

Despite the prevailing bias against herbal treatment in this country, an increasing number of U.S. physicians have begun to experiment with St. John's wort in recent years. Their clinical impressions confirm the results of published literature and paint a picture of a treatment that is substantially effective in real life.

One such physician is Scott Shannon, a psychiatrist in Fort Collins, Colorado. Dr. Shannon was a student of Dr. Andrew Weil and has spent much of his professional career exploring alternative options for emotional illness. In Shannon's opinion, St. John's wort is often effective in mild to moderate depression. "It elevates mood and raises energy, without causing side effects," he says. "Patients tell me they feel brighter, less fatigued, and more able to manage."

He tells the story of Karol, a patient in her middle fifties, who was burdened by numerous responsibilities. "She had lots of irons in the fire," Shannon says. "Young children, aging parents, work stresses—it was all a bit too much for her. She felt chronically depressed and anxious."

Karol tried Paxil, and although she found it helpful, she couldn't tolerate the sexual side effects. Shannon switched her to St. John's wort, and she responded within a few weeks. "She started to wake up with a sense of liveliness she hadn't felt for a while," he explains. "During the day, she felt less glum and had more energy. She also found it easier to manage stress."

Furthermore, all these benefits occurred without side effects. "She tolerated the St. John's wort without any problems," Shannon says. "I very seldom see any side effects with St. John's wort, other than occasional mild stomach irritation."

Besides increased energy and improved mood, my own patients sometimes report normalized appetite, improved sleep, decreased anxiety, reduction in chronic pain, and an increased sense of self-esteem when they start St. John's wort. "When you feel better overall," Shannon says, "it's natural for other symptoms to improve."

Like other clinicians who use St. John's wort, Shannon feels the herb is most appropriate for mild to moderate depression. "St. John's wort is basically a mood elevator and [an] energizer," he says. "It's often my first choice for dysthymia because it works well without side effects. However," he cautions, "it isn't appropriate for major depression, especially if there's a risk of suicide. Drug treatment is better for major depression. Drugs are also better for people with severe and complex psychological trauma, and when there are vegetative signs."

Vegetative signs are the physical symptoms that often accompany major depression, such as slowed speech and movement. These symptoms generally indicate a more severe form of depression, perhaps too severe for St. John's wort.

Are drugs always more powerful than St. John's wort? "Usually," says Shannon, "although they cause more side effects, as well." But there can be surprises. Jacqueline Fields, a family practitioner in Loveland, Colorado, tells the story of an elderly patient in a nursing home who actually did better on St. John's wort than on antidepressant medication.

"Bruce was too depressed to eat well or talk very much to other patients," she says. "He would just lie around most of the time sleeping. We gave him Zoloft, but it didn't seem to do any good. But when we started him on St. John's wort the results were pretty impressive. He got out of bed, ate better, and actually started talking with the other residents."

One of my patients reported a similar experience. "Prozac didn't do anything for me, even after I took it at double doses for three months," she says. "I'm on St. John's wort now, and it's much more noticeable. I have more energy, I sleep better, I worry less, and life seems a whole lot more interesting."

Nonetheless, most clinicians I've interviewed feel that St. John's wort is typically not quite as potent as drug treatment. Its side-effect profile is so much superior, however, that for most cases of mild to moderate depression the herb may be the superior option.

Side Effects of St. John's Wort

Any drug or food supplement can cause side effects in certain people. Actually, foods themselves can be problematic. Milk can cause bloating and diarrhea, cucumbers can cause burping, onions may trigger heartburn, beans usually create flatulence, shrimp can cause severe allergies, and bread may produce the digestive disorder called celiac sprue, to name only a few possible complications of eating. However, St. John's wort is safe and relatively side-effect-free.

In the extensive German experience with St. John's wort as a treatment for depression, there have been no published reports of serious adverse consequences.[17] Even minor side effects are rare. In one study of 3,250 patients taking St. John's wort extract for four weeks, the most common side effect was mild stomach discomfort, and it occurred in only 0.6 percent of patients taking the herb.[18] Allergic reactions such as skin rash and itching developed in 0.5 percent, tiredness in 0.4 percent, and restlessness in 0.3 percent. Other side effects occurred at still lower rates. Only 1.5 percent of the patients dropped out of the study due to perceived side effects, and the total percentage of patients reporting side effects was 2.4.

Among the approximately 1,200 patients observed in St. John's wort versus placebo trials, the overall incidence of side effects was 4.1 percent.[19] (A 19.8 percent side-effect rate is mentioned in the abstract of the *British Medical Journal* overview.[20] However, this is an artificially inflated number, as explained in the appendix.)

Thus, a total of 4,450 patients taking St. John's wort have been screened for side effects. This closely matches the 4,000 patients who received Prozac in premarketing studies (according to the 1997 *PDR*).[21]

Putting all the research together shows that St. John's wort is both safe and effective, according to a level of scientific evaluation that matches what is usually required of drugs. The herb may thus be regarded as a realistic alternative to prescription antidepressants for mild to moderate depression.

CHAPTER SIX

How to Take St. John's Wort

- What is a standardized herbal extract?
- What's the right dosage and form of St. John's wort?
- How much does it cost, and where do I get it?

- Warnings—real and theoretical
- What to expect from treatment
- The big picture

After learning about the benefits of St. John's wort, you are probably ready to know how to take it. The subject is a bit more complicated than it sounds, however, because St. John's wort is an herb instead of a drug; and certain concerns regarding standardization must be explained before I can sensibly provide the appropriate dosage.

When you purchase a drug, you generally know exactly what you are getting. Drugs are single chemicals that can be measured and quantified down to their molecular structure. Thus, a tablet of extra-strength Tylenol contains 500 milligrams of acetaminophen, no matter where or when you buy it.

But herbs are living organisms comprised of thousands of ingredients, and between one plant and another the proportions of all these ingredients may be dramatically different. Numerous influences can affect the nature of a given crop. Whether it was grown at the top or bottom of a hill, what the weather was like, when it was picked, what other plants lived nearby, and what kind of soil predominated are only a few of the factors that can affect the chemical makeup of an herb.

This is one very important reason medical doctors prefer drugs to whole herbs. Conventional medicine tries to deal in standardized, reproducible methods, but with herbs it is difficult to know exactly what you're dealing with.

To get around this problem, modern herbalists often use what is known as a "standardized herbal extract." This is a concentrated form of an herb, "boiled down" until a certain fixed percentage of one or more ingredients is reached. For St. John's wort, biochemists deliberately achieve a fixed proportion of the substance hypericin, the chemical ingredient presumed most responsible for the herb's antidepressant properties. Typical preparations sold in the United States are standardized to contain 0.3 percent hypericin by weight. Such standardization allows a reasonable degree of reproducibility from batch to batch.

It is important to note, however, that the rest of an herb's ingredients are still present in a standardized herbal extract. If you wanted to turn St. John's wort into a drug, you could chemically isolate the hypericin molecule and sell a tablet that contained 100 percent hypericin. Physicians would be much more comfortable with such a form of St. John's wort. They could regard it as a completely repro-ducible treatment and use it like they use other drugs.

However, pure hypericin extract would no longer be an herb. It would be just like all the other drugs manufactured from plants. A standardized herbal extract still retains thou-sands of naturally occurring constituents and still reasonably deserves the designation of "natural." A good analogy is the difference between blackstrap molasses and white sugar. Both are manufactured from sugar cane, but the former is a healthful concentrated extract and the latter a single chemi-cal. A standardized herbal extract is like a carefully prepared form of blackstrap molasses, while a purified hypericin ex-tract would parallel white sugar.

There are two advantages to using a standardized ex-tract instead of a completely purified drug. The first is that there is no evidence that hypericin is the only important or even the most important substance in St. John's wort. Very likely, a combination of ingredients is responsible for the antidepressant properties of this herb.

The second is that many people assume natural sub-stances are more wholesome than drugs. That is hard to prove; nevertheless, many of us prefer to use them instead of chemicals, when possible—a subject addressed at greater length later in this chapter.

There is also one major disadvantage to using standardized herbal extracts: The standardization isn't complete. While two batches of the 0.3 percent hypericin extract will contain nearly identical quantities of hypericin, they may differ substantially in the levels of other important constituents. Thus, doctors interested in reproducibility still have a legitimate concern. A standardized herbal extract is a compromise between achieving quantitative accuracy and sticking close to nature; and like all compromises, it doesn't satisfy either extreme completely.

Dosages

Having explained the complexities of formulating and using standardized herbal extracts, I can now describe the proper adult dose of St. John's wort: 300 milligrams three times a day of an extract standardized to contain 0.3 percent hypericin. Alternatively, some physicians prefer to prescribe 600 milligrams in the morning and 300 milligrams at lunchtime. Due to the occasional side effect of stomach irritation, St. John's wort should be taken with food.

Some St. John's wort preparations list a concentration of 0.15 percent hypericin, and these should be taken in double the dosage just described. Other versions on the market, particularly tinctures, do not list a fixed percentage of hypericin at all. These products may be effective, but the problem of batch-to-batch variability and unknown potency makes them generally less preferable. Finally, several commercial preparations combine St. John's wort with other natural substances believed effective for depression, discussed further in chapter 9. Although there is nothing necessarily wrong with such an approach, I generally prefer targeted treatments to shotgun methods. You simply won't know what is working if you take a pill that contains nine ingredients. Furthermore, combination treatments frequently contain less than optimal dosages of each individual substance.

Dosages for children are discussed separately in this chapter.

How Much Does It Cost, and Where Do I Get It?

St. John's wort is widely available in health food stores, in natural food stores, by mail order, and in some pharmacies. Depending on the form purchased, a typical dosage generally costs from $15 to $25 per month. I recommend staying with a reputable company, such as Enzymatic Therapy, Nature's Plus, Source Natural, Nature's Herb, Yerba Prima, or Nature's Way.

However, even with reputable herb companies, it is still difficult to be sure that you are getting quality product. The FDA closely scrutinizes drugs, but herbs are sold as food supplements and hence receive less careful scrutiny. Consumers may have good reason to wonder whether product labels match actual ingredients.

The supplement industry is averse to being regulated by the FDA because it believes the agency is biased in favor of pharmaceutical companies. This accusation is probably true; yet, the industry has not yet taken any serious steps to regulate itself in lieu of government regulation, which leaves consumers in a bind.

Some supplement manufacturers cite evidence of testing by independent laboratories to verify their claims. Since it is the manufacturer who picks the laboratory, sends the samples, and reports the results, however, it isn't always clear whether such "independent" verification can be trusted completely. Nonetheless, until such time as a truly impartial body comes into being to evaluate the labeling accuracy of supplements, manufacturer-chosen laboratory analysis remains the best method of verification available.

Therefore, I recommend asking for independent testing literature for the particular brand of St. John's wort you are purchasing. Another option is simply to try one brand of St. John's wort, and if it doesn't work, try another.

Warnings—Real and Theoretical

When used in standard dosages, St. John's wort is a thoroughly safe treatment. After years of use in Germany there is not a single published case report demonstrating dangerous drug interactions or toxicity.[22] Nevertheless, numerous books and articles on St. John's wort mention two serious problems as real possibilities: photosensitivity and MAO inhibitor–like reactions to foods. These are highly theoretical risks essentially never observed in practice; but because they are so widely discussed and have frightened some people away from using St. John's wort, I shall explore them at some length.

Photosensitivity?

Certain drugs significantly increase the risk of sunburn. Patients taking sulfa antibiotics, tetracycline, various diuretics, and even tricyclic antidepressants can sometimes develop severe blistering sunburn after relatively short exposure. This potentially deadly phenomenon is called photosensitivity. Patients taking photosensitizing drugs are supposed to stay indoors or, if they must go out, use effective sunblock.

Although physicians seldom give such a warning for the drugs just mentioned, popular articles on St. John's wort frequently make a point of cautioning against sun exposure while taking the herb.

The origin of this concern goes back to the eighteenth century, when light-skinned cattle and sheep grazing on large quantities of St. John's wort were observed to develop severe, blistering sunburn. Ranchers in Oregon and Washington apparently lost millions of dollars of livestock due to sunburn during the "Klamath Weed" infestation of St. John's wort in the Pacific Northwest (as described in chapter 1).

The sun-sensitizing toxin in St. John's wort is the same hypericin listed on standardized extracts of the herb. However, the quantity of hypericin required to cause photosensitivity is believed to be at least thirty to fifty times the recommended dosage.[23]

Photosensitivity has not occurred in a single patient involved in studies investigating St. John's wort as a treatment for depression, nor have any published reports of photosensitivity emerged out of the widespread use of this herb in Germany. A few patients did develop photosensitivity in experiments studying whether St. John's wort could help AIDS patients, but these few cases involved very high doses of synthetic hypericin administered intravenously.[22]

Still, it is always possible that someone might develop sun sensitivity while taking normal oral doses of St. John's wort.

Therefore, for absolute safety, light-skinned people should perhaps stay out of strong sunlight while taking this herb.

MAO Inhibitor–Related Side Effects?

The official German monograph on St. John's wort suggests that patients taking the herb should observe precautions similar to those necessary with MAO inhibitors. However, like the sun-sensitivity issue, this is a highly theoretical warning. I can't find a single published case report of MAO inhibitor–type reactions occurring in patients taking St. John's wort for depression.

As you may recall from the previous chapter, patients on MAO inhibitors must be very careful about what they eat. Cheese, wine, yeast, and other tyramine-containing foods can cause serious, even fatal, reactions. A variety of drugs can trigger the same reaction, including Sudafed, phenylpropanolamine, and other nasal decongestants.

This potential interaction makes MAO inhibitors rather dangerous drugs. The same warning has been associated with St. John's wort, not because such an interaction has ever been observed, but because of one study performed in 1984 that suggested St. John's wort could inhibit monoamine-oxidase.

Subsequent studies failed to substantiate these MAO inhibitor–like effects. As I explained earlier in this chapter, the MAO theory of St. John's wort has fallen into disfavor, to be replaced by a serotonin-based hypothesis. Thus the only basis for fearing MAO inhibitor–type reactions has been essentially refuted. The 1996 *British Medical Journal* review of St. John's wort[25] did not even mention MAO inhibition.

Drug Interactions

Patients considering taking an herb for any purpose commonly ask whether it could interfere with medication they are taking. Since drugs frequently interfere with one another, this is a realistic and sensible concern. Unfortunately, the question is difficult to answer with any certainty.

There are no known interactions between St. John's wort and pharmaceutical medications. However, this statement should not be taken to imply that no such interactions exist. It is certainly possible that unrecognized problems may occur in certain people, because systematic trials have never been performed to look for drug-herb interactions.

Much the same situation exists in the world of drugs. Medical researchers do not go down the list of available drugs and try them in every possible drug combination. It would be too expensive and time-consuming, and deliberately exposing patients in clinical trials to unnecessary medications would be unethical, as well. Drug interactions are usually discovered by accident or by analogy with already discovered drug interactions.

What can be said for certain is this: In the extensive German experience with St. John's wort, no reports of problems caused by the simultaneous use of St. John's wort and a pharmaceutical drug have ever been published.[26]

Long-Term Effects

Another question people often ask about herbs is whether it is safe to take them for many years. This is a legitimate concern because many drugs cause problems that only become evident after a long period of use, and herbs could conceivably do the same thing.

Unfortunately, there has never been a study formally evaluating the safety of St. John's wort over a period exceeding eight weeks. Wide usage in Germany over the last ten years has failed to reveal any delayed harmful effects, but this does not mean that there couldn't be hidden, subtle, or occasional side effects that simply haven't yet been noticed. Thus, it is impossible to make a definitive statement that St. John's wort is safe over the long term.

The same lack of knowledge prevails for Prozac, other antidepressants, and indeed virtually all medical therapies. The only absolutely foolproof way to determine whether or not long-term harm exists would be to take two identical populations, give one half the drug and the other half placebo, and keep the experiment going for decades. If after fifty years or so no problems cropped up in the treated group, one could then conclude that a treatment was absolutely safe in the long run.

Obviously, such an experiment has never been done, whether for drugs, herbs, vaccinations, food preservatives, or foods. Thus, the long-term safety of all treatments must be regarded as not established.

Some people feel that because St. John's wort is a natural herb it is more likely to be safe in the long run than a drug, but this is more of an emotional statement than a rational one. Numerous herbs have been shown to be potentially toxic, including comfrey and chaparral. For that matter, fatty foods appear to be carcinogenic. In other words, there is no guarantee that St. John's wort is safe just because it's natural.

Is St. John's Wort Safe During Pregnancy and While Nursing?

Like answering the question of long-term risks, establishing safety during pregnancy and while nursing is very difficult. Drug companies are reluctant to state that any drug can be used safely during pregnancy and nursing because there is no way to be sure without trying it; and that may run unacceptable risks. The same may be said for St. John's wort. Although there is no evidence that this herb should be avoided during pregnancy and nursing, no absolute statement as to its safety can be made, either.

Is St. John's Wort Safe for Children?

Yet again, this is a question that can't be answered with certainty. All the studies of St. John's wort were performed with adult patients. Much the same situation exists for Prozac. Nonetheless, Prozac is frequently used for children, and St. John's wort may be appropriate, too.

Most practitioners who prescribe St. John's wort for children lower the dose proportionately by weight, using 130 pounds or so as the average adult weight. Thus, a 65-pound child might be given one-half the normal adult dosage.

Additional Warnings

St. John's wort is not appropriate treatment for severe, major depression, as previously noted. Most of the scientific studies of St. John's wort evaluated its effectiveness in mild to moderate depression (HAM-D scores of 24 or less). In the opinion of clinicians who use it, St. John's wort should not be relied upon for the treatment of severe depressive symptoms because its effects do not seem to be strong enough.

Major depression is a dangerous illness, where the risk of suicide is always present. In such cases, medically supervised use of antidepressant drugs may be lifesaving (although this remains unproved).

St. John's wort may also not be appropriate treatment between major depressions for patients who suffer from frequent major depressive episodes. While research indicates that continuous antidepressant drug treatment can prevent recurrence, St. John's wort is probably not powerful enough to provide the equivalent benefit.

Finally, symptoms resembling depression can be caused by a wide variety of medical illnesses, including low thyroid conditions, anemia, and asthma. It is important to exclude such gross physical causes of depression before turning to self-treatment with St. John's wort.

What to Expect from Treatment

Although every person is different, St. John's wort commonly produces a gentle, gradual elimination of many of the symptoms of mild to moderate depression. The nature of these benefits is not fully captured by the rigid language of medical terms. Therefore, actual descriptions by people who have found St. John's wort useful are provided here.

One of the most common statements I hear is that people feel energized and revivified, but without speediness or jaggedness. As one young woman said, "It's more like the energy of a good night's sleep than a cup of coffee."

However, this increase of energy occurs so smoothly you may not be able to notice it right away. Some people only recognize that they've been feeling more energetic when they stop taking St. John's wort and subsequently sink back to their former state of fatigue.

"I had forgotten what it was like," a thirty-seven-year-old man said three weeks after quitting the herb. "I didn't think it was working at all, but once the St. John's wort wore off I started to sleepwalk through my day again." When he took it the second time, he was looking for the change and noticed it at once.

St. John's wort can also improve the ability to stay alert, think clearly, concentrate, and cope with stress and other distractions. The following description given by a forty-three-year-old mother of two captures some of these effects. "It used to be, after three hours at work I was ready to take a nap," she said. "I couldn't concentrate on my tasks, and all the numbers I was supposed to enter into reports seemed to blur together. But on St. John's wort, I don't get tired till about three in the afternoon, and then it's no more than what anyone else feels. And when I get home I still have energy to spare for my children."

A thirty-year-old magazine editor put it this way: "I feel less scattered. It's like I have a better capacity to put my mind on task. Previously, I'd sink into a state of half-alert confusion, like my thinking was going one way and another at the same time. St. John's wort gives me enough extra mental energy to take charge of my own mind and make it do what I tell it."

St. John's wort can also improve energy levels indirectly. As an example, exercise is one of the best ways of increasing energy, but when you're depressed, you may find it difficult even to start. St. John's wort can help you to break this vicious cycle and improve your lifestyle, which will in turn provide additional benefits.

Besides enhanced energy, patients who find St. John's wort helpful also typically report a lightening or elevation of mood. It isn't like a drug high, nor the almost mechanical happiness that some people say they experience on Prozac. Rather, it seems to most closely resemble the buoyancy of spirits that goes along with a normal good mood.

"I feel more playful now," one twenty-seven-year-old auto mechanic told me. "Instead of sinking down into a kind of drudgery, which is my normal state way too often, I want to have fun. At work I joke around with the other guys more, and at home I don't just sit around turning my problems over and over in my head. I get out and do stuff I like."

Another patient expressed his experience with St. John's wort this way: "It lifts my head out of the clouds. Although I don't usually get extremely depressed, I'm vaguely blue and down most of the time. I get by all right but I always seem to be unhappy about something. St. John's wort makes a big difference with that. Not that I don't ever get unhappy—I still do—but it isn't a constant thing. I go up and down more, instead of hugging the down side."

Another patient described this effect as "increased emotional energy." He said that St. John's wort "not only makes my mind feel more alert, it helps me feel more strongly. Before I used to feel kind of numb and disconnected. On St. John's wort I get more excited, more involved with life."

In similar fashion to its effects on energy, St. John's wort elevates mood gradually. A typically cited figure is four to six weeks. However, a German physician and author of an influential text on St. John's wort suggests giving the herb even more time to work. Dr. Rudolf Fritz Weiss says, "The mood lightening effect does not develop quickly—it is necessary to give the drug [St. John's wort] not just for weeks, but probably for two or three months."[27] However, he goes on to say that "the first effects will usually be noted after two or three weeks."

Because the energizing and mood-elevating properties of St. John's wort occur without stimulant side effects, this treatment is often quite useful for depression accompanied by mild anxiety. As one patient said, "Because I have more emotional energy, and I'm less gloomy, anxiety-provoking thoughts don't have as much power over me as they used to."

St. John's wort is not a tranquilizer, but by alleviating depression without producing artificial stimulation, it may produce a net effect of decreased anxiety. Dr. Weiss recommends combining St. John's wort with mild herbal tranquilizers for additional benefit, as described in chapter 10.

Many patients who take St. John's wort also report an improvement in sleep quality. Like the other effects of St. John's wort, this effect is gentle and "grows on you." After some period of taking the herb, many patients state that they sleep more soundly and restfully.

"I seem to go deeper," a twenty-three-year-old college student told me. "Before I used to hover near the surface most of the night, still processing my classes and turning my assignments over and over in my head. Now I feel like I go all the way under more of the time."

St. John's wort does not directly induce sleep. The improvement in sleep quality appears to follow elimination of depression. In those cases when St. John's wort fails to alleviate depression (and it certainly doesn't always succeed) sleep doesn't seem to improve either.

A similar connection also probably accounts for St. John's wort's positive influence on eating habits. People whose depression manifests as lack of desire for food frequently report improvement of appetite with the herb. This effect may be most notable in elderly patients. One seventy-year-old woman told me that when she started taking St. John's wort "food seemed to have more of a taste."

Depression can manifest as irritability rather than unhappiness. The daughter of the woman I just mentioned states unequivocally that "St. John's wort makes my mom a lot less grouchy. She doesn't get mad all the time."

Again, since St. John's wort is not a tranquilizer, this reduction of irritability is probably directly related to the alleviation of depression. The same effect is commonly seen with chemical antidepressants as well, although the side effects of drugs in the Prozac family can worsen appetite loss.

Self-esteem and ability to tolerate risk may also improve with St. John's wort. Taking the herb may also reduce shyness. The effect is seldom "miraculous," as sometimes claimed for Prozac, but is nonetheless definite. Once more, St. John's wort's direct effect on depression seems to be at root.

As one man in his late twenties said, "Now that I have energy and feel fairly cheerful, I'm not so afraid to show my face in public. Before I didn't have much confidence that anyone would want to see me. I wouldn't have wanted to see me—I was always depressed. It's not like I've turned into Billy Crystal or anything now, but I feel like I have the inner *oomph* to get out there better."

The fact that St. John's wort is a natural herb plays a big role in some people's experience with it. For them, taking an herb *feels* much more acceptable than depending on a drug. "I hate being dependent on Prozac" is a comment I have heard dozens of times. "I feel like I'm some kind of sick person who needs medicine when I take drugs. It's an awful feeling," a thirty-seven-year-old carpenter said of her experience with Prozac. "But I don't mind taking St. John's wort. It's like taking a vitamin, or eating granola. It's a positive experience instead of an embarrassing one."

"Herbs are meant to be used for healing," another patient said. "Animals eat herbs when they don't feel well, too. It's a natural thing to take them, but Prozac isn't natural."

This attitude toward St. John's wort is based on feelings and intuitions, rather than cold facts. Those who do not share the underlying attitude often don't understand why herbs should be different from drugs. Doctors, for example, often tend to scoff at the notion of "natural." They point out that many drugs come from herbs, too.

While this is true, none of the chemical antidepressants come from herbs. They are all synthetic single chemicals. And St. John's wort, with its rich mixture of naturally occurring ingredients, simply feels more wholesome to people for whom that matters.

"I'm an environmentalist, too," said one of my patients. "I believe in sticking closer to nature whenever I can. I buy all cotton—I'd never dream of wearing polyester clothes. Taking an herb fits in with my lifestyle better."

Just because something is natural, however, doesn't mean it's perfect. St. John's wort doesn't always succeed. Some people take it and feel no improvement at all. (The same thing happens with Prozac, of course, and more often than its reputation might suggest!) Others may think they feel an improvement and then decide after a while that it was wishful thinking.

For example, a thirty-eight-year-old physician colleague of mine tried St. John's wort and other alternative treatments for a full two years in what proved to be a vain attempt to treat his depression naturally. He frequently told me, "I think it's working now—I seem to be on an upswing," using the exact same words so often it finally became a joke. When he finally tried Zoloft, the results were dramatic and indisputable. "I was just hoping it would work before," he said. "Zoloft is helping me in a way that I don't have to pinch myself to believe it."

Of course, Zoloft doesn't always work, either. It's not easy to come up with a figure on how often St. John's wort is beneficial for mild to moderate depression, but my guess would be somewhere between 50 and 75 percent. As I said in the note to the reader, this is a useful herb, not a miracle cure. It's a good tool for treating depression, and one that can satisfy the desire for "natural" treatment. However, it's not the last word on the subject.

Don't Forget to Treat the Whole Person

We are a pill-happy society, and to substitute St. John's wort as a natural pill instead of a chemical one is to miss a large part of the picture. Illustrating this point very well in *Listening to Prozac*, Peter Kramer states on page 292, "The patients I medicate with Prozac tend first to have undergone extensive courses of psychotherapy. . . . There needs to be a readiness for Prozac, [which] works best in patients whose conflicts are resolved but whose biologically autonomous handicaps remain."

In other words, if a person has done his or her psychological work, but remains held back by moods that seem connected to built-in brain chemistry, the use of a drug (or herb) may be helpful. But pills shouldn't be used as the sole and single remedy for depression.

Many of us suffer from complex and stubborn emotional binds that cannot be simply alleviated by taking a substance. Rather, it is often necessary to tease apart these constrictions, to loosen their grip, and to soften their imperious domination. It takes a skillful and sensitive psychotherapist to accomplish this, not a tablet.

Yet for some people, even years of excellent psychotherapy fail to relieve depression. They seem prey to moods that have a life of their own, as much physically built-in as brown hair or blue eyes.

We don't really know for sure whether mild to moderate depression is genetically inheritable. It may be that depressive habits of mind are passed along just like mannerisms or figures of speech. If all members of a family tend to say "please" when they don't understand something they've heard (like everyone on my wife's side), we don't attribute this shared habit to DNA. We understand that they all simply learned the habit together.

Similarly, depression may be to some extent learned by imitation. Children may notice parental patterns of unhappiness and adopt them for their own. But in some people it appears that genetics must play a role. No matter how hard they try to compensate or cope, no matter how many bad emotional habits they solve through psychotherapy, depressive moods prevail. These are the people who find antidepressant therapy most helpful; and St. John's wort may be helpful for them, too. Still, such treatments work best after the hard work of psychotherapy has been completed.

Besides psychotherapy, there are many other common-sense aspects of depression that shouldn't be neglected in favor of antidepressants. I already mentioned the necessity of excluding physical diseases that may masquerade as depression, such as low thyroid. It is also important to consider basic lifestyle issues.

Poor diet can certainly increase symptoms of depression. There is a strong clinical impression, and at least some double-blind evidence, that in some people caffeine and sugar can produce symptoms of depression.[28] Numerous vitamin and mineral deficiencies can cause depression, as well. Low levels of folic acid, vitamin B_{12}, pyridoxine, iron, and magnesium are some of the most commonly implicated nutritional influences on depression.

Besides diet, other lifestyle issues can make a significant impact on depression. Exercise, enjoyable activities, a comfortable living situation, satisfactory employment, tolerable levels of stress, and good relationships with friends and family are all important.

I remember one thirty-year-old woman who had tried both antidepressants and St. John's wort without success. Her depression lifted only after she left her mother's home and moved into her own house. Interestingly, this solution was suggested, not by her therapist or myself, but by her seven-year-old niece!

People sometimes tell me that they have tried common-sense changes and received no benefit, so they went back to their former lousy lifestyle. I often suggest revisiting the issue. With the additional help offered through the use of

St. John's wort, solutions that were previously attempted without results may become more effective. The same may be true of psychotherapy: The mood and energy boost of an antidepressant, whether natural or otherwise, may facilitate progress.

I will return to this subject in chapter 10. For now, I will just say that the best approach to treating depression (and addressing any other problem) is to look at the whole picture. Taking into account medical, psychological, and lifestyle issues, St. John's wort may make an important contribution to a comprehensive solution.

CHAPTER SEVEN

How St. John's Wort Compares with Drug Treatment

- Direct comparisons
- Indirect comparisons
- What clinicians say
- Side-effect comparison
- An interesting discrepancy
- Safety
- Subtle details

The preceding chapter showed how St. John's wort has been proved effective in the treatment of mild to moderate depression. The studies from which this conclusion is drawn are scientifically sound, involve reasonably high numbers of patients, and are published in reputable journals.

However, none of the studies quoted in the last chapter directly compared the effectiveness of St. John's wort against pharmaceutical options. This chapter explores the question: Which is the more appropriate treatment for mild to moderate depression, St. John's wort or antidepressant drugs?

Direct Comparisons

In 1993, E. Vorbach and colleagues performed an experiment designed to compare the effectiveness of St. John's wort and imipramine in the treatment of mild to moderate depression.[29] Imipramine is the oldest of the tricyclic drugs, and it is used relatively seldom in present clinical practice because of its many side effects. Its efficacy has never been surpassed, however, and imipramine remains the "gold standard" against which newer antidepressants are usually compared.

For example, when Eli Lilly was trying to get Prozac approved, the company sponsored extensive clinical comparisons between their new medication and imipramine. The results did not show that Prozac was more powerful than imipramine. Rather, all they demonstrated was a comparable effect, which was sufficient for the FDA.

Vorbach chose to compare St. John's wort against the same gold standard. He and his fellow researchers prepared tablets of St. John's wort extract that were identical to imipramine in appearance, flavor, and consistency. Patients were then randomized into two groups, one receiving 300 milligrams of standardized St. John's wort three times daily and the other receiving 25 milligrams of imipramine three times daily. A total of 135 patients at twenty separate physicians' practices were enrolled in the study and followed for six weeks. The age range was eighteen to seventy-five years, and male and female patients were included in about equal proportion.

Using the HAM-D depression index, physicians rated patients' levels of depression at the beginning of the study and at two-week intervals until the end. Patients' levels of depression were also monitored with a separate scale known as the Clinical Global Impressions scale (CGI). This scale allows a somewhat different perspective on the progress of depression. The recorded progression of these scores provides a direct comparison between the antidepressant powers of imipramine and those of St. John's wort.

At the beginning of the study, HAM-D scores for both groups of patients averaged about 20. Patients treated with St. John's wort improved their scores by 55 percent, while those taking imipramine only improved by 45 percent. At the end of the test, 81.8 percent of the patients on St. John's wort were rated as "significantly improved" according to the CGI, while only 62.5 percent of the patients on imipramine received that score.

Because the differences between these numbers were not large enough to be statistically significant, the study's conclusion was this: St. John's wort and imipramine are equally effective in the treatment of mild to moderate depression. Since imipramine is known to be as effective as Prozac, it seems logical to assume that St. John's wort would prove as effective as Prozac if they were matched head-to-head, too.

Unfortunately, there is a serious flaw in this otherwise excellent piece of research: The dosage of imipramine was too low. Participants received 75 milligrams of imipramine daily and no more, while in real clinical practice doses of 150 to 250 milligrams are frequently necessary to achieve optimum results. One study that compared imipramine to Zoloft and placebo settled on an average dose of about 200 milligrams of imipramine per day.[30] In other words, the 75 milligrams used for this St. John's wort comparison study may simply have been too low to display imipramine's full powers.

The researchers knew they were using a low dose of imipramine. Actually, they chose it deliberately to keep the double-blind structure of the study intact. Imipramine causes a number of significant and obvious side effects, such as dry mouth, dizziness, and sedation, and the higher the dose the stronger the side effects. In comparison, St. John's wort produces next to none. If Vorbach had used imipramine in full doses, participants receiving the drug instead of the herb would almost undoubtedly have been able to guess which group they were in. The examining physicians would also have been able to figure it out, and the whole purpose of the double-blind set-up would have been negated.

Furthermore, the researchers backed their dose choice by citing a standard German textbook of drug therapy for psychiatric illnesses, which states that 50 milligrams of imipramine should be adequate for most outpatients. However, most physicians in the United States would not agree. A mere 75 milligrams of imipramine a day seems subtherapeutic by U.S. standards, making the study appear ludicrous instead of impressive.

A similar trial (with a similar flaw) was performed by G. Harrer and colleagues in 1993.[31] It compared the effectiveness of St. John's wort against that of another tricyclic antidepressant: maprotiline. Maprotiline is an interesting antidepressant for two reasons. Unlike most tricyclics, it is a highly specific drug. It elevates levels of norepinephrine but does not change serotonin at all. This makes it the opposite of Prozac, which raises serotonin without affecting norepinephrine. Maprotiline is also unusual for its unusually rapid onset of action. Most people who take it experience a reduction in symptoms of depression after only a week or two, compared to the typical four to six weeks most other antidepressants require.

Harrer's study enrolled 102 patients at six doctors' practices and followed them for four weeks. The patients were both male and female and ranged in age from twenty-four to sixty-five years old. On average, their initial HAM-D scores were about 21, representing moderate depression.

Half the patients were given St. John's wort and the other half maprotiline. The HAM-D rating was then repeated at the end of week two and week four. As expected, maprotiline was the early leader, producing more marked improvements at the first retest. However, by four weeks St. John's Wort had fully caught up with maprotiline's benefit. In both groups, the final improvement in HAM-D scores was essentially the same: about 50 percent.

Nonetheless, there was one significant difference between patients given St. John's wort and those treated with maprotiline. According to the CGI, a higher percentage of patients taking the herb were evaluated as "very much improved" or "no longer ill" compared to those taking the drug. The researchers felt that this difference was probably due to the side effects caused by maptrotiline.

Once again, while the results were impressive, their validity is undercut by the low drug dosage used in the study. Participants received only 75 milligrams of maprotiline a day. In normal clinical practice, this is only a starting dose for the drug. Physicians usually push the level upwards to achieve optimum effects. A typical final dose might be 100 to 150 milligrams daily.

Again, a drug was unfairly handicapped in its competition with St. John's wort, making the study's results questionable. In reviewing the imipramine and maprotiline studies, the *British Medical Journal* expressed a wish that "the comparator should be tested in therapeutic doses" and refused to take the results seriously.[32]

As previously noted, it isn't clear how this problem could be solved. If any study were to use full doses of antidepressant drugs, many patients would be able to guess that they were taking them and not the herb, and the double-blind would be broken. A completely different approach is needed, but none have yet been developed. In the final chapter of this book I suggest some possible approaches.

Indirect Comparisons

There is another way to evaluate the relative effectiveness of St. John's wort and drug therapy: compare the drop in HAM-D scores that each treatment produces in its own separate trials. Such a method resembles comparing runners' times when racing alone. Direct head-to-head competition defines the winner more conclusively, but individual records can be used to qualify potential competitors for the real match. Similarly, cross-study comparisons can show whether St. John's wort is a realistic contender.

To ensure this comparison is between apples and apples, not apples and oranges, all studies described below used the same seventeen-item HAM-D test in their evaluations of results. I focus here on trials involving the newer antidepressant drugs because those are the ones most frequently prescribed for patients with mild to moderate depression.

One Prozac study evaluated 372 patients with mild depression (HAM-D scores of 15 to 19), but the results were not very impressive.[33] Placebo-treated and Prozac-treated patients experienced essentially identical improvements in HAM-D scores. In other words, Prozac proved on average to be no more effective than a sugar pill for treating mild depression.

Faced with these negative results, the authors of the study resorted to questionable statistical manipulations in what seems to be a desperate attempt to prove Prozac effective. They looked closely at the responses of each individual patient and identified a subgroup that responded well to Prozac. Their conclusion was that Prozac is definitely effective for certain patients with mild depression and not others.

Actually, this form of statistical reasoning is highly dubious. If two contestants are pitching pennies and come to a draw, it's always possible to pick out a few selected tosses and say, "Contestant two was much better with certain pennies than contestant one." Such a statement really communicates nothing except to reiterate the normal action of the laws of chance. A draw is a draw, even if there are a few brilliant tosses along the way.

Thus, Prozac's mediocre results in this study suggest that it is not a terribly effective treatment for mild depression. A comparable study of St. John's wort in treating mild depression showed much better results.[34] In this trial of 105 patients with HAM-D scores averaging about 16, participants were given either St. John's wort or placebo. Patients receiving St. John's wort demonstrated an average improvement rate almost twice as high as for those taking placebo.

This evidence appears to suggest that St. John's wort is effective for a broader spectrum of mildly depressed patients than Prozac is. However, this comparison cannot be taken as scientifically solid, because the patients in the St. John's wort group were not identical to those in the Prozac study. One difference was that the St. John's wort patients were chosen on the basis of older, looser definitions of depression than the relatively rigorous *DSM* criteria that the Prozac researchers used. Also, one trial was conducted in Germany and the other in the United States. Numerous cultural and demographic differences may thus confound the results.

Another relevant study followed a total of 416 outpatients with average HAM-D scores of about 13.[35] Patients were randomly assigned to receive either Zoloft, imipramine, or placebo. Both the Zoloft- and imipramine-treated groups showed a statistically significant response to treatment, and the results were quite similar to what was achieved by St. John's wort in the study just described.

However, once again, differences in patient population weaken the power of this comparison study, as well. The situation is analogous to runners from different countries establishing records in their own homeland, under different conditions of weather, altitude, and terrain. Numerous subtle factors make a precise comparison of speed impossible. Nonetheless, what *can* be said for certain regarding treatment of mild depression is that St. John's Wort is definitely a contender.

It is more difficult to find drug studies to compare against St. John's wort studies for patients with *moderate* depression. While most of the research into St. John's wort concentrated on moderately depressed patients, the Eli Lilly company was unable to provide me with studies that evaluated Prozac in a similar population. The best I could do was to find a study that evaluated patients with moderate depression when they were given either placebo or the tricyclic drug desipramine.[36] The results showed a success rate of 55 percent.

This figure is exactly the same as the overall effectiveness of St. John's wort when results of all studies of the herb are combined.[37] Thus, for both mild and moderate depression, St. John's wort seems at least roughly comparable to drug treatment.

St. John's wort hasn't been studied for patients with severe depression (HAM-D scores of 25 or higher). This reflects the widespread impression among practitioners who use St. John's wort that the herb isn't effective for those who are severely depressed.

What Clinicians Say

The research just described, while suggestive, is far from definitive. To flesh out a picture of the relative power of St. John's wort and drugs, let's now turn to the clinical impression of physicians familiar with the herb.

In his official German monograph on the subject, Dr. Rudolf Weiss says, "The antidepressant effect [of St. John's wort] is not so unequivocal and intensive as those of modern synthetic antidepressants."[38]

This view is shared by other clinicians who use St. John's wort. Dr. John Motl, a psychiatrist with extensive experience in alternative treatments, told me that St. John's wort is milder in its effects than Prozac. "I wouldn't use it for major depression," he said. "But in mild to moderate depression it can be very helpful."

Based on my own experience, I would agree. I have seen several patients attempt to self-treat severe depression with St. John's wort, but none were successful. In each case, chemical antidepressants proved significantly more effective.

Even though St. John's wort is weaker than drug treatment for serious depression, this doesn't mean that it is comparatively less effective in mild to moderate depression. The studies described in the previous section seem to suggest that the benefits are roughly equal.

Nonetheless, many physicians believe that even in mild to moderate depression drugs are more powerful than St. John's wort. This is Scott Shannon's impression, the Colorado psychiatrist I mentioned in the previous chapter. "Drugs are usually stronger," he says, "but I frequently try St. John's wort first because of the better side-effect profile."

My own experience suggests that Prozac and similar drugs are a bit more potent than St. John's wort for mild to moderate depression. Patients who try antidepressant medications seem to report dramatic results more often than those that use the herb. However, I'm not sure I trust my own impression. We may all be under the influence of the power of suggestion.

My own evaluations may have been subconsciously affected by the media hype over Prozac. Do I—and Scott Shannon and others in the medical field—unconsciously expect superior results from drug treatment and thereby convey more confidence to our patients when we prescribe medications? Does this same bias also skew our informal evaluation of patient improvement? I'm not sure.

Mild to moderate depression is such a fluid and subjective illness that it leaves plenty of room for the power of suggestion to act on both doctors and patients. The entire situation is murky. Some patients may respond to the fame of Prozac and experience especially positive results because they expect to experience them. The effect can go the other way, too, however. Some of my patients distrust drugs on general principle and are loathe to accept that they might ever receive benefit from one. Since they are far more comfortable with natural herbs, this emotional bias might very well affect their response to treatment.

Perhaps this is why St. John's wort is the antidepressant of choice in Germany. There, both physicians' and patients' attitudes are strongly sympathetic to the use of herbal medications and less impressed by the power of drugs. St. John's wort may benefit from a topspin of positive feeling in Germany, just as Prozac does on this side of the ocean.

The double-blind study was developed by medical researchers in order to eliminate the effects of suggestion. If the true identity of treatment or placebo is concealed from both physicians and patients, the results should be more reliable. When it comes to antidepressant drugs, however, the usual precautions may not be sufficient. For, as previously explained, the obvious side effects of drugs may "break the blind" and allow patients and doctors to determine which is drug and which is placebo.

In chapter 4, some of the potential confusion caused by this disintegration of the double-blind structure is discussed. Psychologists Roger Greenburg and Seymour Fisher further explore the magnitude of this effect in an article that attempts to evaluate the true effectiveness of Prozac.[39] They suggest that all double-blind trials need to take into account the side effects of drugs and their influence on results. But they do not suggest any definitive way to accomplish this.

Besides helping patients know whether they are taking drugs or placebo, side effects throw another monkey wrench into the works by turning drugs into "active placebos." This term refers to the following phenomenon: When a drug produces demonstrable symptoms, even unpleasant ones, its ordinary power of suggestion may be enhanced. You might say, "Since I have a dry mouth and my heart is racing, I know I'm taking a powerful drug." Some authorities have recommended using drugs such as antihistamines instead of sugar pills for placebo, to balance out this particular form of the placebo effect.

However, St. John's wort has a strike against it in this regard. It's so gentle, you might come to the conclusion that it can't possibly be doing anything. This is precisely what happened in the case of my patient Laura (described at the beginning of chapter 6). Laura was absolutely certain St. John's wort couldn't be working for her because she didn't feel lousy when she took it! This impression actively blocked her awareness of its genuine effects.

Finally, the precise nature of side effects can influence the perceived effectiveness of a treatment. Prozac's stimulating qualities are especially useful in this regard because they may mimic recovery from depression. Any stimulant, even a cup of coffee or a candy bar, can produce a temporary uplift in mood. Similarly, Prozac's stimulant effects can create an illusion of improvement and enhance the placebo effect.

In the preceding paragraphs, I've listed at least six forms of the power of suggestion. They may all play a role in confounding our evaluation of the relative effectiveness of

St. John's wort versus chemical antidepressants. Further research may demonstrate that St. John's wort is actually just as powerful for mild to moderate depression as any drug—*if* the uneven effects of suggestion are removed.

Without doubt, some patients definitely respond better to St. John's wort than to drug therapy. Two such cases were mentioned in chapter 5. While I was working on the present chapter, a sixty-year-old woman came to my office and told me a third such story. St. John's wort had proved more effective for her than Prozac, Effexor, or MAO inhibitors. I won't be surprised to see many more such cases in the future. Questions of suggestion aside, St. John's wort has definitely been shown to be an effective treatment for mild to moderate depression. Whether it is slightly less powerful than, equally powerful to, or even possibly more powerful than drugs for this condition remains to be seen.

Side-Effect Comparison

In almost all studies of St. John's wort, the incidence of side effects is extremely low. As described in the last chapter, one trial of 3,250 patients given St. John's wort showed a total side-effect rate of only 2.4 percent.[40] The most common reported problem was stomach distress (0.6 percent), followed by allergic reactions (0.5 percent) and tiredness (0.4 percent).

This large study was not blinded. When all the double-blind trials comparing St. John's wort to placebo are lumped together, the observed incidence of side effects attributed to St. John's wort is 4.1 percent.[41] This is still far lower than the incidence of side effects attributable to antidepressant drugs.

Tricyclic antidepressants produce side effects in virtually everyone who takes them. The newer antidepressants are better, but they are still far more prone to side effects than St. John's wort. According to the 1997 *PDR*, 10 to 15 percent of patients taking Prozac develop so much anxiety, nervousness, or insomnia that they are compelled to quit taking the drug. The incidence of sexual side effects may be as high as 30 percent or more.[42] One German study showed an overall Prozac side-effect rate of approximately 19 percent, which is about five to eight times greater than the occurrence rate with St. John's wort.[43] This particular figure may be especially meaningful because, like the St. John's wort studies cited, it involved German observers and patients and thus compares apples and apples.

Another way to look at the question is to examine the rate at which people discontinue medications due to adverse effects. Approximately 31 percent of patients given tricyclic antidepressants quit taking them because of side effects.[44] The numbers with Prozac seem to be somewhat lower, perhaps around 17 percent,[45] although the exact number remains a matter of controversy. In comparison, only 1.5 percent of patients taking St. John's wort discontinue due to side effects, according to the 3,250-patient drug-monitoring study just mentioned in the preceding text.

These stark differences in side effects make a compelling case for trying St. John's wort before resorting to drugs. The 19 percent frequency of side effects caused by Prozac represents an immense quantity of human suffering, considering the millions of people taking the drug. This suffering would be substantially reduced if St. John's wort were more widely used.

An Interesting Discrepancy

The St. John's wort side-effects figures cited here were derived from the combined results of the 3,250-patient drug-monitoring study and the St. John's wort versus placebo studies. Nevertheless a few studies report much higher percentages of side effects. The origin of these inconsistent results demonstrates yet another fascinating example of the placebo effect.

In the St. John's wort versus imipramine study discussed earlier, a full 12 percent of the patients taking St. John's wort reported side effects, the most frequent being dry mouth and dizziness.[46] This is three times or more the total incidence of side effects reported in other studies, and remarkably close to the 16 percent of patients who developed side effects on low doses of imipramine. It is important to note as well that dry mouth and dizziness were also the predominating imipramine side effects.

Another significant fact is that while the numbers were close, the perceived intensity of side effects was quite different in those taking the herb versus those taking the drug. Nearly all patients on St. John's wort said their side effects were mild, while for those on the low doses of imipramine, seven out of twenty-two patients complained of moderate to severe side effects.

Nonetheless, one may ask why these side effects for St. John's wort occurred at all? Dry mouth was not even an issue in the trial of 3,250 patients, and dizziness occurred at a very low rate of 0.15 percent. Why should dry mouth and dizziness suddenly show up in high percentages when St. John's wort is being compared to imipramine? This bizarre change deserves an explanation.

Fortunately, it's not hard to find one. Imipramine is a drug famous for causing dry mouth and dizziness. When taken in full doses, it causes dry mouth in virtually all people and dizziness in a high percentage. What we are probably seeing here is a kind of shadow effect caused by suggestion. Patients in a double-blind comparison between drug and herb *think* they may be taking a drug and thus develop some of the side effects they expect from the drug—even when they're not taking it.

A confirmation of this explanation may be found in drug versus placebo studies. Patients given placebo typically develop side effects at remarkable levels when they think they may be taking a real drug. For example, in the Zoloft-imipramine-placebo study cited earlier, 17 percent of the patients taking placebo reported dry mouth and 16 percent reported dizziness.[47] The same kind of shadow effect is at work here.

Thus, the high rates of side effects seen in St. John's wort versus drug tests are probably falsely inflated. The 2.4 to 4.1 percent rate discovered in all other studies is much more likely to be correct.

Safety

Side effects and safety are slightly different issues. One refers to annoying problems, the other to the risks of serious injury or even death. For example, MAO inhibitors may give you insomnia as a side effect, but if you eat the wrong foods while taking them you might die. Similarly, tricyclic drugs will almost certainly make your mouth dry. However, if you accidentally take as little as four times the recommended amount, you may end up in the hospital with seizures, heart injury, dangerously low blood pressure, or even coma. Many depressed patients prescribed tricyclics have used them to commit suicide.

The Prozac family of drugs is far safer than either MAO inhibitors or tricyclics. Patients have taken as much as 100 tablets at a time with no worse result than agitation and vomiting (although there have been a few reports of more serious injury). This safety factor figured extensively in Prozac's early advertising campaign. As one drug rep said in recommendation of his product, "Even if it doesn't work, your patient won't be able to kill himself with it."

St. John's wort is also quite safe. Although many millions of people have taken it in Germany, no serious adverse effects have been recorded. Studies involving physical exam and serial blood tests have never shown any measurable effects.[48] Photosensitivity and MAO inhibitor–like side effects are sometimes mentioned as risks, but as discussed in the previous chapter, the latter probably does not exist at all and the former only occurs with doses far higher than normally prescribed.

Nevertheless, firm statements about long-term safety cannot be made for either St. John's wort or any pharmaceutical antidepressant. In chapter 4, I explained how such a determination would require difficult studies that would take many years. I also described a particular concern regarding Prozac: that it may cause long-term injury analogous to tardive dyskinesia, the distressing and permanent movement disorder that occurs in some people who take antischizophrenic drugs.

While this risk remains speculative, Scott Shannon thinks that it is a realistic enough basis for limiting the use of Prozac in mild to moderate depression. "I think we need to be very careful about prescribing drugs that dramatically change brain chemicals," he says. "We don't really know all the ramifications. I wouldn't like to give Prozac to someone with mild to moderate depression and find out later that I've caused some kind of long-term harm."

Of course, it is possible that St. John's wort could cause long-term harm as well. But since it doesn't produce as dramatic changes in brain chemistry as Prozac, it is reasonable to suspect that the herb may be relatively safer when taken for an extended period of time.

Psychological Safety

Another safety issue with regard to use of antidepressants refers to psychological rather than physical risks. This type of potential harm from using Prozac and other antidepressant drugs is seldom mentioned but may pose a danger as serious in its own way as outright chemical toxicity.

Those who depend on Prozac for psychological well-being may experience a subtle but damaging distortion of self-image. "I need drugs to be normal," goes the unspoken refrain, and it is a damaging message that may cause real harm. Children prescribed Prozac may be the most susceptible to this subtle harm because their developing identities may permanently incorporate this sense of dependence on an artificial substance.

In contrast, St. John's wort gives a completely different and far more wholesome message. Psychologically speaking, it "feels" more like a food than a drug; it is a natural plant rather than a synthetic chemical. This emotional point is usually disregarded by physicians, who have difficulty recognizing the problem because their profession makes them perfectly comfortable with drugs.

Increasingly, Prozac has been offered as a treatment for mildly depressed children. But, considering this point, I question whether it is always worth the risk. Chronic dependency on a drug may do psychological damage that outweighs the good produced by relief of depression. If there were no other choice but to use Prozac, physicians and parents might deem that risk warranted. However, since St. John's wort represents an effective and more psychologically wholesome alternative, it may be a preferable option. (Please note that neither Prozac nor St. John's wort has been fully evaluated for its benefit in treating children.)

Does St. John's Wort Produce Exactly the Same Effects on Depression As Antidepressant Drugs?

There is still one more level of comparison between St. John's wort and drug antidepressants that should be considered. Amidst all the HAM-D values and formal evaluation criteria, the inward nature of depression, and recovery from it, includes many indefinable experiences that could be significant. Emotional suffering is beyond the crude grasp of rating scales. It would be like trying to measure the extent of good character or the depth of gratitude.

This is an area that eludes science and moves into the realm of literature and poetry. While a writer might fill hundreds of pages detailing a person's inner life and still fail to capture it completely, a seventeen-item HAM-D can't possibly come close.

It is for this reason that, even when two antidepressants produce similarly measured changes in depression, their actual effects may be quite different. Peter Kramer speaks of different layers, or levels, of depression, some of which tricyclic drugs seem to "touch," others of which seem more accessible to Prozac. St. John's wort may touch areas of the mind unique to itself.

Actually, each antidepressant drug probably produces its own characteristic effects on depression; and if language could easily describe such differences, more people would talk about it. The best descriptions I've heard came from two unusually expressive patients. Their communication skills have given me a glimpse of these largely unrecognized distinctions.

"Prozac turns on an 'outgoing' button in me," says Caroline, a forty-year-old freelance writer. "I find myself talking to people in a more assertive, pushy way, almost without even noticing. It's as if Prozac pushes a switch and turns me into an extrovert. I like not being depressed, but I don't always want to feel the way Prozac wants me to feel."

Caroline has tried other antidepressants, too, and rates them differently. "Wellbutrin doesn't push the extrovert button. Instead it turns up the 'contrast' dial, increasing my mental clarity. I can think more clearly, organize myself better, and get more things done. I become an effective workaholic instead of an aggressive party animal. On Wellbutrin, I *like* cleaning house, which says a lot. However, my feelings seem shoved way in the background."

She's also taken Serzone. "Now that's a really different medication. It makes me moody and dreamy and languid. The moods are happy and the dreams are interesting. However, I feel so dreamy that I don't talk to people or get anything done."

Caroline puts St. John's wort in its own class. "What St. John's wort does for me is to put me in a bouncy mood, what they used to call a sanguine disposition. I feel carefree, light, and even a bit euphoric. It doesn't make me as assertive as Prozac, as organized as Wellbutrin, nor as dreamy as Serzone, but it feels more normal."

Another patient, whom I shall call Jim, says that he finds Prozac very gentle. "It doesn't give me any side effects," says this fifty-six-year-old civil servant. "All I notice when I take it is that I don't waste my time second-guessing myself. I make my decisions and carry them through without obsessing over them. I feel more myself on Prozac."

But Jim appreciates St. John's wort, as well. "I also feel more myself on St. John's wort but it's a different 'self.' The herb doesn't stop me from chewing things over in my mind, like Prozac does, but it does stop me from getting tied up in knots about it. You could put it this way: Prozac turns me into a shoot-from-the-hip John Wayne kind of guy, while St. John's wort makes me more like Gregory Peck. You know, the calm, reflective type. I'm not sure which I like best."

This type of thoughtful analysis belongs to a larger discussion about the nature of personality and the appropriateness or inappropriateness of using substances to modify it.

Certainly, there is no reason to believe that anyone else will experience antidepressant treatments in exactly the same ways that Caroline or Jim does. My purpose in mentioning their descriptions is not to dictate how you'll feel, but simply to show that there are many personal details that must be taken into account.

CHAPTER EIGHT

How to Decide If St. John's Wort Is Right for You

- Checklist of symptoms
- Other indications for St. John's wort
- When not to use St. John's wort

Among patients who visit family practitioners' offices, depression is far more common than high blood pressure, according to at least one study.[49] It is a prevalent and largely undertreated illness. Every year, at least 15 million Americans experience major depression, and the number who experience chronic depressive symptoms of a mild to moderate nature is undoubtedly even higher. Depression costs society tens of billions of dollars. In addition to their direct health care costs, people who are depressed miss more work than the rest of the population and experience five times the rate of disability.[50]

More important than any dollar figure, however, is the fact that depression causes a tremendous amount of human suffering. According to one study, the loss of well-being and physical capacity caused by depression typically exceeds the negative effects of diabetes, back pain, and arthritis.[51] It decreases the ability to enjoy life, impairs child-rearing, cramps social relationships, interferes with healthy lifestyle habits, and inhibits career success. Furthermore, depression's vague symptoms frequently cause extended and aggressive medical examinations and testing.

There is no question that Prozac and other antidepressant drugs have improved the lives of many depressed people. But the fear of these drugs' side effects has kept many people from seeking treatment.

St. John's wort's ability to treat the symptoms of mild to moderate depression without side effects makes it a potentially superior choice to conventional drugs for many millions of people. However, despite its long use in Germany for that reason, most people in the United States do not know whether St. John's wort is a realistic option for them.

Mary's story illustrates this common situation. When she came to see me this year, the first words she said were, "My doctor wants to put me on Prozac. According to him, the reason I'm so tired all the time is that I'm depressed. I thought I was anemic, but he says not."

From what I knew of Mary, I agreed with her doctor's assessment. Her close friend had called me just before the appointment. "Mary's always unhappy, exhausted, and worried," she had said. "She doesn't eat right, and even though the doctors say there's nothing wrong with her, she always complains that something hurts. She gets by all right, and she's definitely not suicidal, but she's sure not having a lot of fun."

Mary looked a lot older than fifty-two. Weariness was written on her face; and after I had looked at her for a while I felt like taking a nap. Although I agreed with her family physician's assessment that Prozac would probably help her, Mary didn't want to take Prozac. She'd had many bad experiences with drugs in the past. "I always seem to get reactions to medications," she said. "I get rashes, stomachaches, and headaches when no one else does. I guess I'm just sensitive. What I want to know is whether I could take St. John's wort instead."

She'd raised the subject with the other doctor, too. Although he'd said he was open to the idea, he'd confessed that he knew nothing about it. I questioned Mary closely about her symptoms and soon concluded that she would be a perfect candidate for treatment with St. John's wort. She responded even better than I'd hoped. After three months, she looked ten years younger.

Mary was a good candidate for St. John's wort because she fit the picture of mild to moderate depression. Her symptoms of depressed mood, fatigue, sleep disturbance, appetite disturbance, anxiety, and multiple small physical discomforts spoke of classic chronic depression. But for several reasons, it seemed she wasn't suffering from a severe major depression: She was coping with life successfully, she wasn't suicidal, and her primary care doctor had only suggested she take Prozac, rather than insisting on it. Thus, St. John's wort was just right for her.

As I mentioned in chapter 2, dysthymia is the psychological diagnosis that fits most closely with what I'm calling mild to moderate depression. Dysthymia has an official definition, and I've designed a checklist (see table 8-1) based roughly on its criteria, but modified slightly to focus on those symptoms for which St. John's wort seems most frequently effective.

Table 8-1
Symptoms of Mild to Moderate Depression Checklist

Primary Criteria:

☐ *Do you chronically feel depressed?*

or (especially for children and adolescents)

☐ *Do you seem unusually irritable?*

Plus Two or More of the Following Secondary Symptoms:

☐ *Do you feel constantly tired, whether physically or mentally?*
☐ *Do you suffer from insomnia?*
☐ *Are you easily overwhelmed?*
☐ *Are you frequently anxious?*
☐ *Do you have difficulty concentrating?*
☐ *Does depression interfere with your appetite?*
☐ *Do you experience many small physical discomforts?*

If you have one of the primary criteria listed above and two or more of the remaining criteria, you may benefit from St. John's wort (as long as your symptoms are mild to moderate, and not severe).

If you are not severely depressed but you satisfy the terms of this checklist, St. John's wort is definitely worth trying. Of course, it might not prove effective. No treatment works all the time. But your chances of good results with St. John's wort are about 50 to 75 percent.

The remainder of this chapter provides detailed explanations of these checklist questions, carefully distinguishing between mild to moderate and severe symptoms. Also, it touches on a few additional indications for St. John's wort as well as reiterates those circumstances in which St. John's wort is definitely not an appropriate treatment.

Primary Symptom: Do You Experience Depressed Mood?

Depressed mood usually manifests as a chronic sense of unhappiness, glumness, and melancholy, although for some people, numbness and apathy are better descriptions. In major depression, this mood is overwhelming, unbroken, and often excruciatingly painful; but if your depression is mild to moderate, your unhappiness is not as intense, you have both good and bad days, and most of the time your suffering seems more troublesome than disabling.

St. John's wort is an effective mood elevator in mild to moderate depression. Patients taking it typically say they feel brighter, more enthusiastic, and better able to cope with life.

Randy, a forty-three-year-old small business owner, is a good example of this effect. When he first came to me, he said he made a decent income and spent quality time with his wife and children, but he always felt that he was struggling. Although he had been in therapy for several years, his mood hadn't improved in all that time.

"Something inside me is always pulling me down," he said. "Every night I get gloomy for no reason and have to turn on music or call a friend to make it go away. I know the same thing can happen to anyone, but it happens way too often for me. A day doesn't ever seem to go by when I'm not fighting depression."

I felt that Randy was a good candidate for St. John's wort. He was clearly depressed, but because his symptoms came and went every day I didn't think his level of depression was too severe. Also, I noted that he was able to fight off his gloom by working at it. In classic major depression, such depressed mood is typically overwhelming, unrelenting, and more intense. Randy was coping with life effectively and could enjoy himself much of the time. I suspected that St. John's wort could deal with his symptoms easily, and I proved to be right.

"I'm a whole lot less moody," he said after two months of taking the herb. "Don't get me wrong, I still have my down times. But the up and the down are a lot more balanced. Life's a lot more fun."

Randy had tried Prozac before, but it made him impotent. "This herb doesn't cause the same problem. Everything's great in that department."

Actually, Randy's depression fell on the mild side of the mild to moderate scale. St. John's wort can successfully treat depression more severe than Randy's. However, it has its limits. Lucy is a good example of what St. John's wort can't do.

This thirty-three-year-old retail clerk came to my office requesting St. John's wort, but she went out with a prescription for Prozac and a referral to a psychiatrist.

Lucy was tearful from the moment she walked in, and her story further showed me the depths of her depression.

"I try to think positive," she said, "but I feel so hopeless and worthless. I've even thought of taking my husband's hunting rifle and shooting myself." After she said this, she burst into tears.

It didn't take me more than about five seconds to recognize that St. John's wort was not for Lucy. Constant crying, overwhelming feelings of worthlessness and guilt, and, most especially, frequent and realistic thoughts of suicide mean that depression has gone too far for St. John's wort.

I explained to Lucy that she had fallen too deeply into depression to benefit from herbal medicine. "St. John's wort isn't strong enough," I said. "You need something like Prozac, and I want you to see a psychiatrist this afternoon. I'm afraid you're going to hurt yourself otherwise."

As for many others in the depths of major depression, Lucy found dramatic relief through antidepressant drugs, and the medication may have saved her life. Fifteen percent of patients who suffer from major depression commit suicide. Although it's difficult to find hard evidence to show that antidepressants actually reduce the incidence of suicide, it certainly seems that they do. Drug treatment seldom fails to produce a dramatic turnaround in severe major depression, and suicidal thoughts are often one of the first symptoms to improve.

Although St. John's wort is ideal for mild to moderate depression, drug treatment is the best option for severe depression.

Alternate Primary Symptom:
Do You (or a Loved One) Seem
Unusually Irritable?

In most cases, depressed mood is the primary sign of mild to moderate depression. However, excessive irritability or social withdrawal can sometimes appear instead. This variation of depression occurs especially often in children, adolescents, and senior citizens.

I recall one ten-year-old who developed an extremely short fuse shortly after his parents divorced. Even after a year of useful psychotherapy this symptom wasn't getting any better. Michael would start a Lego project and then tear it apart as soon as he encountered the slightest flaw. If his pet dog barked too much, he'd scream and hurl childish insults. He'd also get annoyed with his friends—even his best friends—and stalk to his room and shut the door on them when they were visiting. Pretty soon Michael didn't have any best friends.

None of this behavior was like him. Michael had previously been a sensitive but even-tempered child. Wracked with guilt, his divorced parents wondered what they should do. Ultimately, a psychiatrist who specialized in alternative medicine prescribed St. John's wort for their son, along with a few other natural treatments (as described in chapter 10), and within two months he had returned to normal.

Like other antidepressants, St. John's wort may be quite helpful when depression shows up as irritability. I've seen similar results with senior citizens who grew increasingly irascible and withdrawn after an illness or following the death of a spouse. It is especially attractive for the very young and the very old because of its favorable side-effects profile.

Do You Feel Constantly Tired, Physically or Mentally?

A general feeling of tiredness, sleepiness, and exhaustion is a common symptom of mild to moderate depression. People suffering from severe depression often can't even get out of bed, but in mild to moderate depression tiredness is a problem, not a master. You may wake up tired and find that exercise fails to give you a boost, and whether it's work or play, all your activities are hampered by a chronic feeling that you just don't have enough energy.

St. John's wort can be an effective energizer in mild to moderate depression. It often produces a gradual but sustained increase in physical, mental, and emotional energy. As one patient said, "I used to be running on fumes, but now I feel like I have gas in the tank." Both work and play may become easier and more enjoyable when you have enough oomph to carry them through with enthusiasm.

Nonetheless, St. John's wort is not a stimulant. It's effects are very specific: Only those whose fatigue is caused by depression experience increased energy. Its energizing effect is also very smooth, entirely lacking the jagged edge of Prozac. However, make sure not to give up too soon. Improvement may take a month or more to manifest.

Do You Suffer from Insomnia?

Insomnia is a classic symptom of depression. Apparently, whatever imbalance in brain chemicals is directly caused by depression, that same imbalance interferes with sleep.

Successful treatment of depression usually improves sleep as well.

The typical pattern of depression-induced insomnia is early morning awakening. However, difficulty falling asleep and restlessness during sleep may also occur. Inadequate sleep may contribute to fatigue, moodiness, and difficulty coping with life.

In whatever way insomnia manifests itself, St. John's wort can be beneficial. And because of its low rate of side effects, this herb can sometimes be a better treatment for depression-related insomnia than chemicals. Drugs in the Prozac family frequently worsen insomnia, and the older drugs typically produce excessive sedation. St. John's wort is a "clean" antidepressant that affects sleep only by addressing the underlying problem.

St. John's wort is not a direct sleeping pill, as its results take many weeks to develop. More potent sleep-aids may be necessary for severe insomnia.

Are You Easily Overwhelmed?

Being easily frazzled by stress is another symptom of mild to moderate depression. What other people find merely unpleasant, you may find almost impossible to manage. The multiple demands, interruptions, and irritations of work and family life may seem overwhelming. If you were in a severe major depression, they really would overwhelm you, and you'd probably fail to manage them altogether. But in mild to moderate depression you cope, yet only by working a lot harder than you feel you should need to.

Although it certainly isn't a "magic" cure, St. John's wort may provide just enough boost to make normal life stresses easier to deal with. Patients have told me they experience increased reserve capacity and a greater ability to stay calm in the midst of many demands. And because it doesn't cause anxiety or sedation, there is nothing to counteract this direct benefit.

Are You Frequently Anxious?

Like insomnia, anxiety seems to be linked to depression at a fundamental, brain-chemical level. Although the precise connection remains unclear, researchers suspect that the two symptoms must be connected because antidepressant drugs frequently alleviate anxiety as well. (This is an example of "listening" to drugs.) Even drugs in the Prozac family can reduce anxiety in the long run, although they often worsen anxiety symptoms at first.

The anxiety of mild to moderate depression can be pervasive, annoying, and continuous. You feel that you are always on edge, always expecting something bad to happen. You don't seem to be able to relax like other people, and you wish your nerves would simply take a vacation. However, these symptoms are less intense than the severe, almost disabling anxiety that may accompany major depression.

St. John's wort is often effective for the anxiety associated with mild to moderate depression. As one patient said, "I feel distinctly calmer. I can deliberate over decisions without getting all worried. Loud noises don't startle me the way they used to, and when I try to relax I can actually get there."

St. John's wort is not sufficient treatment, however, for severe anxiety. Recently, a physician called me up wanting me to talk her patient out of taking St. John's wort. "She's highly agitated," the physician said. "She scans the room when she's in my office, wakes up at night with panic attacks, and her husband says she paces back and forth at dinner."

I agreed that St. John's wort was not the right approach for this patient. It would be too mild and too subtle. She probably needed quick-acting drug medication. Intense anxiety requires more aggressive treatment than St. John's wort can provide. Even for relatively mild anxiety, many alternative physicians combine a natural antianxiety treatment with St. John's wort to enhance and speed effectiveness, such as described in chapter 10.

Do You Have Difficulty Concentrating?

In recent years, *attention deficit disorder*—called by its initials, ADD—has become a household word. Both adults and children are now frequently diagnosed with this syndrome, whose symptoms include difficulty concentrating, easy distractibility, and lack of ability to prioritize tasks. Similar symptoms can occur in depression.

Antidepressant drugs sometimes alleviate such problems, both in those who are depressed and those with ADD. Unfortunately, the side effects of such drugs can be counterproductive. Many antidepressant medications seem to hamper short-term memory, interfere with linear thinking processes, and generally make people feel scatterbrained. Since St. John's wort produces none of these awkward side effects, it may be a preferable choice for ADD-like symptoms in depression. It may also be useful for ADD itself.

Does Depression Interfere with Your Appetite?

Loss of appetite is another common symptom of depression. It occurs most frequently in the elderly but can occur in anyone, especially those whose temperament might be described as chronically anxious or high-strung. St. John's wort is frequently effective against this symptom. It is not an appetite stimulant and doesn't cause weight gain in normal people, but the herb often normalizes eating as it eases depression.

If loss of appetite reaches serious proportions or is accompanied by alarming signs of severe depression, pharmaceutical treatment is preferable. A medical workup to rule out physical causes of appetite loss may be necessary as well.

Do You Experience Many Small Physical Discomforts?

Another classic symptom of depression is multiple, relatively minor discomforts that shift from place to place. Known technically as somatic symptoms, headache, palpitations, and wandering muscle pain are some of the most frequently cited problems. Some researchers have suggested that serotonin levels play a role; however, the exact connection between depression and physical discomfort remains murky.

Pharmaceutical antidepressants sometimes relieve these physical manifestations of depression. A study reported in 1994 showed that St. John's wort can do so as well.[52] In this trial, thirty-nine patients whose depression included somatic symptoms were treated with either St. John's wort or placebo. Even patients taking placebo improved (as usual!), but those given the herb improved significantly more.

One of the most dramatically improved symptoms was muscle pain. At the start of the study, eight patients in the St. John's wort group complained of generalized discomfort and aching. At the end, only two continued to report those symptoms. The response to placebo was negligible: Out of an initial twelve patients complaining of muscle pain at the beginning of the study, ten still complained of symptoms after taking placebo for four weeks.

Headaches also decreased markedly in the St. John's wort group, dropping from nine to two. Patients given placebo again showed a poorer response, dropping down from eleven only to seven. St. John's wort was significantly more effective than placebo for heart palpitations, sleep disturbances, and fatigue as well.

Although small, this study suggests that St. John's wort is an effective treatment for depression with somatic symptoms. Clinical experience further corroborates the results. For example, I remember a patient named Thiu who had been in a relatively minor automobile collision two years before she came to see me. She had received excellent care for her injuries, including physical therapy, chiropractic, massage, and osteopathy. Nonetheless, she still complained of aching shoulders, arms, legs, hip, back, and neck.

None of her physicians could find anything wrong. Neither her family practitioner, chiropractor, osteopath, physical therapist, or massage therapist could identify a single lingering problem that would explain her pain. The chiropractor ultimately concluded she was depressed and referred her to me for possible treatment with an antidepressant.

When I saw Thiu, I immediately agreed with the chiropractor's diagnosis. I approached the subject gingerly, however, because no patient who hurts wants to be told "it's all in your head." I first asked her to describe what had happened in her own words.

Thiu explained that ever since the accident she'd felt tired, anxious, and unhappy. "I was already stressed out when I was rear-ended," she said, "and that was the last straw."

Her answers to my questions soon assured me that depression was at least one of her problems. I expressed my suspicions as tactfully as I could, pointing out that anyone as hurt as she had been might become depressed. "And depression can make healing more difficult," I concluded.

Rather reluctantly, Thiu agreed that it could be possible, but she didn't believe in taking drugs. Her family practitioner had made the suggestion months before, and she had refused. "I don't want to take pills," she said. But when I told her that it was only St. John's wort that I was suggesting, she gave me a big smile. She was perfectly happy to try a natural herb.

After four weeks of taking St. John's wort Thiu felt dramatically better. "I think I went to the chiropractor about six months longer than I had to," she said; and the chiropractor wholeheartedly agreed. He had been trying to get her to consider antidepressants for at least that long.

In Thiu's case, depression seems to have played a significant role in the maintenance of her chronic symptoms. There are many other possible causes of chronic pain, of course, including subtle soft-tissue injuries, but depression is frequently an aggravating factor. For this reason, St. John's wort may be worth a try in many instances of chronic pain.

Other Indications for St. John's Wort

Besides the symptoms listed above, there are a few other indications that St. John's wort might be useful. These are situations that aren't listed in any formal criteria but frequently arise in real life.

Have You Tried Psychotherapy but Reached a Plateau?

I am a great believer in the value of psychotherapy. In my opinion, a good therapist can help alleviate many lifelong problems and facilitate self-awareness and receptivity to change. The benefits may last for the rest of your life. Of course, not all therapists are skillful, and therapy is sometimes considered a notorious waste of time. But more often than not psychotherapy proves distinctly useful, especially for depression.

Nonetheless you may have found that therapy helped you for a while, and then it stopped making a difference. Perhaps you feel that you have a remaining level of depression that's more biological than psychological in origin. Another possibility is that chronic depression may be reducing your ability to make important life changes. It is precisely in these circumstances that antidepressants can make a significant contribution. And in many cases St. John's wort may be even better than drugs.

Have You Been Prescribed Pharmaceutical Antidepressants for Mild to Moderate Depression?

Since the advent of Prozac, physicians have been dispensing antidepressant drugs to people with mild to moderate depression. If you are one of these individuals, you may wish to consider switching to St. John's wort in order to reduce side effects. There's no reason to endure sexual dysfunction or insomnia while trying to feel better. St. John's wort may very well prove equally effective and much more pleasant.

If you are taking a drug for severe depression, however, such a switch should be undertaken cautiously, if at all. St. John's wort is not powerful enough to keep severe depression in check.

Perhaps the only time when St. John's wort is appropriate for major depression is if you are getting ready to stop drugs anyway. For example, your last major depression may have been several years ago, and your doctor says it would be OK to try tapering off. Since the alternative is taking nothing at all, transitioning to St. John's wort certainly couldn't hurt.

Nevertheless, if severe major depression is part of your history, please be careful! Make sure you have the support of friends and family and you remain supervised by a professional. Major depression is a dangerous illness.

When Not to Take St. John's Wort

The warning symptoms of severe major depression include greatly decreased interest in normal activities, severe anxiety, severe insomnia, pronounced agitation or slowing down, overwhelming feelings of worthlessness, obsessive preoccupation with guilt, inability to cope with life, and most especially, significant suicidal thinking. St. John's wort is definitely not appropriate if you experience symptoms such as these. It is too gentle and gradual in its effects. I'd recommend taking medications, and soon.

St. John's wort is also inappropriate treatment for obsessive-compulsive symptoms or depression with psychotic features (such as hallucinations and delusions). Finally, don't take St. John's wort for generic symptoms such as fatigue without first getting a good medical checkup to rule out underlying disease.

If your symptoms of depression are troublesome but manageable, and they are not due to any underlying physical illness, St. John's wort may very well be an ideal first choice for you.

CHAPTER NINE

Working with Medical Doctors and Alternative Health Practitioners

- Working with medical doctors
- Why physicians are so often prejudiced against herbs
- Why the FDA doesn't approve herbs as treatments for medical illnesses

- How to interest your medical doctor in St. John's wort
- Working with doctors of osteopathy (D.O.s)
- Working with other alternative practitioners

I n many places, this book has stressed the risks of severe major depression and the necessity for conventional medical treatment when symptoms pass a certain level of intensity. I've also pointed out that a thorough medical checkup may be essential to rule out the possibility of physical disease masquerading as symptoms of depression. For these reasons, a knowledgeable physician makes an ideal partner to help individuals interested in taking St. John's wort for depression.

Unfortunately, few physicians know much about St. John's wort, and many even view it with considerable suspicion. This can be a real, practical obstacle to obtaining expert guidance. Although you can choose instead to visit alternative practitioners, who may be quite familiar with the herb, they may not be sufficiently well versed in the medical side of the equation. This chapter suggests strategies for working effectively with conventional physicians and also explains the pros and cons of utilizing various alternative health professionals instead.

Working with Medical Doctors (M.D.s)

In the course of a phone conversation with a local psychiatrist, I recently had the opportunity to experience physician prejudices against St. John's wort. We started out talking collegially about a mutual patient. When I happened to mention that I was writing a book on St. John's wort, however, the conversation suddenly came to a halt.

"You're writing a book on what?" he said, after a long pause.

"The herb St. John's wort," I replied. "You know, the herbal antidepressant that's getting in the news."

After another pause, he said, "Oh, yes, I remember. Another doc told me it was a safe placebo."

"Actually, it's not just a placebo, Bob," I said. "The German studies on it are quite strong. It really works."

"Aren't they pretty lax about their research there?"

"Germany's not exactly a third-world country. But anyway, the *British Medical Journal* recently published an impressive review of the literature." I knew this would get his attention. U.S. physicians respect the *British Medical Journal*, probably because it's written in English.

"Really. Well do you think it does some good?"

"Definitely. For mild to moderate depression, anyway. Not for major depression."

"So it's a useful homeopathic then?"

"Not homeopathic, Bob. It's a standardized herbal extract."

A homeopathic treatment is a preparation that involves dilutions so extreme not a single atom of the original substance is left. What Bill was trying to do when he compared St. John's wort to homeopathy was to "damn it with faint praise." Homeopathy is regarded as a bad joke by nearly all medical doctors in this country.

"Now I remember, Steve," he said. "I read the other day that it's an MAO inhibitor. Sounds like dangerous stuff."

It took me several minutes to work through the MAO-inhibitor myth.

Next, he complained that the German trials were too short. "What does a six-week study prove?" he asked. When I reminded him that the qualifying studies for Prozac only lasted four to six weeks, he attacked the size of the studies instead. "Only 1,750 patients in the trials? Isn't that a bit small?"

I pointed out that most drugs are approved after studies are completed on 1,000 to 2,000 patients, many of whom do not complete the full study period. I then had to reassure him that the St. John's wort studies were double-blinded (probably more successfully than most drug studies), that they used formal HAM-D scores instead of "vague impressions," and that side effects had been fully evaluated in over 4,000 people.

It took about twenty minutes to give my colleague a realistic understanding of St. John's wort. Still, I don't think I ever convinced him. This didn't surprise me, because most M.D.s in the United States are heavily prejudiced against herbal treatments.

The reasons for this ingrained distrust are complex and involve historical, cultural, and practical issues. It is always easier to work with people when you understand their way of thinking. For this reason, I explain these motivations in some depth.

Why Physicians Are Prejudiced Against Herbs

When conventional medicine was first taking shape, about 400 years ago, herbal treatment had been the prevailing standard of care. But to the way of thinking of these early medical physicians, traditional herbal medicine had several strikes against it. First, it was the province of women—and conventional medicine was a male profession. Also, while these doctors wrote in Latin and Greek, herbalists lacked higher education, which made herbal medicine seem to belong to the lower class. Finally, medical doctors were busily adopting the newly developing principles of science, while herbs remained a folk tradition. Medical doctors put herbology in the category of superstition.

In an attempt to distance themselves from herbal traditions, physicians turned to chemical medications instead. Mercury and arsenic were some of the first of the popular new treatments. This proved to be a great misfortune to many people, who would have been much better off taking either herbs or nothing at all, but it was the harbinger of modern pharmaceutical medicine.

This conflict and separation occurred during the fifteenth through eighteenth centuries. Nonetheless, the old antipathy toward herbs lingers today. Few doctors think about it consciously. However, at a subconscious level the very notion of treating diseases with herbs seems archaic and unscientific to them. The public's newfound interest in herbs looks to doctors like a revival of ancient ignorance.

Of course, many drugs were originally derived from herbs, though most are now synthesized. Digitalis, quinine, Sudafed, codeine, guaifenesin (an expectorant), and theophylline are only a few of the many medications that were initially extracted from plant sources. But there is a significant difference between drugs extracted from herbs and the herbs themselves.

The constituents of whole herbs are complex and highly variable, and altogether "too natural" for physicians' comfort. Pharmaceutical manufacturers use chemical techniques to extract single active ingredients from plants and sell them as purified drugs. Because these extracts are quantifiable, reproducible, and completely analyzable, they fit well within the culture of Western science. Whole herbs do not.

This focus on a single active ingredient represents a fundamental philosophical change from the attitude of old-fashioned herbalists. The village herb woman believed that

God made herbs for the express purpose of healing illnesses and naturally assumed that everything in the herb was important. But medical scientists take a materialistic view. According to them, medicinal plants evolved their active ingredients either by accident or as an evolutionary strategy to poison herbivores who might otherwise eat them. Physicians expect to find a single important chemical constituent in individual herbs, reasoning that the chance of there being two lucky accidents in a single herb is small. This single substance is the drug; and the whole herb is viewed as nothing but raw material. Scientists don't share the ideal of "natural medicine" and can't take seriously the notion that whole herbs might be better than purified drugs.

Medical schools do not address the subject of herbal medicine, except to add a quaint historical flavor to lectures or to describe the efforts of pharmaceutical companies to scour the rainforests for new plant sources of medications. It's always drugs that physicians are interested in: purified chemicals. If these chemicals are extracted from plants, it is not objectionable, but it is not a recommendation either. Synthetic "designer drugs" engineered for a certain biochemical purpose are much more thrilling.

This is a philosophical and cultural divide that isn't easy to cross. The concept of the standardized herbal extract (as described in chapter 6) reassures medical physicians to some extent. Nonetheless, they still distrust herbs and remain legitimately concerned about reproducibility between batches. Doctors would always prefer a single purified chemical if given the choice. St. John's wort extract, because it contains innumerable substances, still seems too "fuzzy." (Interestingly, vitamins are far more acceptable to medical doctors because they themselves are purified chemicals.)

Besides cultural and historical obstacles, there is one more important reason that physicians don't use herbal medicine: The FDA doesn't license herbs as treatments for specific illnesses. Herbs can only be sold as food supplements without specific health claims. The cause of this situation is a fascinating subject in its own right.

Why the FDA Doesn't Approve Herbs As Treatments for Illnesses

It is a standard belief in alternative medicine that there is a conspiracy between drug companies and the FDA to keep herbs inaccessible. "They know how effective they are," goes the argument. "They're afraid that if people used herbs, drug profits would go down."

While there is no question that the FDA has too cozy a relationship with drug companies and that drug companies enjoy reaping profits whenever they can, these are not the reasons herbs fail to be licensed. The real explanation is far less thrilling than a massive covert conspiracy.

The FDA is composed to a great extent of scientists who share the cultural prejudices of physicians. Rather than believing that herbs are stunningly effective and therefore dangerous to drug company profits, they instinctively feel that herbs are archaic, probably ineffective, and useful only as raw material for chemical drugs. Herbs do not loom up as a threat; rather, they seem beneath notice.

However, even if an herb such as St. John's wort does prove effective, there is still a special and particular reason it can't become an approved treatment in the United States.

This has to do with the flow of money behind research. The FDA drug approval process is very expensive. It begins with animal safety studies, then moves on to human safety studies and analysis of the drug's distribution and elimination in the human body. Next, controlled studies are performed on small numbers of patients. Finally, so-called phase III trials begin, verifying the benefits and risks of the drug in large numbers of patients (generally 1,000 to 2,000). Strict experimental design and reporting must be upheld, special conferences must be held at every step of the process, and researchers from numerous medical centers must be recruited. Only after about five or six years of such study can a "New Drug Application" be submitted to the FDA.

The purpose of this lengthy process is to avoid disasters like thalidomide. However, these legitimate hurdles raise costs to $200 million per drug or higher. The drug company that holds the patent on a drug can afford to risk such enormous sums, because it can recoup the expense through sales. But an herb can't be patented. If one company paid for the research that it took to get an herb approved, other companies could reap the profits by selling it.

Pharmaceutical manufacturers can't be criticized for failing to throw away $200 million per herb. They're not charities—they're businesses. I don't see many alternative practitioners expending their personal life savings on research into herbs, either.

Money spent on herbal research is money that can never be recovered, and that kind of money is always scarce. Only grants from the government (or extraordinary benefactors) fit into this category, and this is a relatively small and competitive pool. Furthermore, research into herbs doesn't rank as a top priority. High tech approaches seem to be much "sexier" than the perceived backwater of herbal medicine.

For all these reasons, U.S. research into nonpatentable substances is typically limited to puny trials involving twenty-five or fewer patients. This reality is often turned on its head and used as "evidence" that herbs are basically "unscientific." Actually it indicates more about the financing of research than about the value of herbs themselves.

Presently, most of the good research on herbs is performed in continental Europe, where herbal medicine occupies a higher rung on the status ladder. Physicians prescribe herbs, the government endorses them, and general funding for basic herbal research is far more available. The consequence is that a great deal of the best evidence for the effectiveness of herbal treatments comes from European countries.

Unfortunately, U.S. physicians seldom read European medical journals, because they aren't written in English. Many physicians even assume that European studies are somehow no good. This presumption is absurd, of course—the European Union has unified regulations for the approval of drugs, and they certainly meet acceptable scientific standards. There is really a kind of xenophobia at work here. American physicians typically respect Australian and British studies, although there is nothing intrinsically more scientific about their research than what comes out of Germany or France. The real obstacle seems to be nothing more than language.

In the final chapter of this book, I recommend strategies to initiate a workable herb approval process in the United States. Until such time as my suggestions are implemented, however (and don't hold your breath), most medical doctors will probably remain uncomfortable working with herbs. It may be up to you to impress on your physician that St. John's wort is a respectable treatment.

How to Interest Your Medical Doctor in St. John's Wort

Because of all of the obstacles discussed, it can be quite a challenge to persuade doctors to take St. John's wort seriously. The job must be approached carefully and thoughtfully. It is important to know at the outset that physicians are *not* impressed by stories, testimonials, and anecdotes. For this reason, *Beat Depression with St. John's Wort* may not make the best impression on your doctor! I've attempted to paint a picture of how St. John's wort works by telling stories, but to a physician this will probably seem like an excessive reliance on untrustworthy evidence.

Physicians look for hard data. And although such information is included in chapters 5 and 7, these chapters also include numerous stories that will distract physicians from the main point. Therefore, a summary of the most important research on St. John's wort, presented in a format that most physicians should find acceptable, is included in the appendix to this book. Feel free to copy those pages and take them to your doctor.

You also may wish to present copies of actual published scientific trials. Some of the most impressive effectiveness research is detailed in the August 1993 *British Medical Journal* article and the Hansgen study.[53,54] For side effects, the 3,250-patient drug-monitoring study will be the most informative.[55] This study is also useful because it counters a false impression given by the abstract to the *British Medical Journal* article: that St. John's wort causes side effects in 19.8 percent of those who take it. (I explain the fallacy behind this figure in the appendix.)

You can obtain reprints of these articles for a reasonable charge from the Herb Research Foundation, 1007 Pearl St., Suite 200, Boulder, CO 80302. Their phone number is (303) 449-2265.

Many physicians will be reasonably receptive to receiving such information from their patients. However, a few doctors still cling to an authoritarian stance and may decline to take seriously anything a mere patient brings to their attention. If this is your experience, I suggest changing doctors. Such posturing no longer has an acceptable place in modern society.

"Alternative" Medical Doctors

A relatively small number of medical doctors define themselves as "alternative," "complementary," or "holistic." Like myself, they may incorporate a variety of unconventional methods into their practices. Nearly all physicians of this type will be quite familiar with the use of St. John's wort. Unfortunately, I can't make a blanket recommendation that such physicians will satisfy your needs.

Many alternative medical physicians are responsible, prudent, intelligent, and careful practitioners. They provide medical care at a high standard of excellence and choose only the best of the alternative options. Physicians of this type may be your best possible option.

It is my sad experience, however, to have observed that a number of unconventional medical doctors do not function at an acceptable level. Some seem indiscriminate in their acceptance of alternative techniques, while others appear to be motivated entirely by a desire to maximize profits. You have to be quite careful when you choose an alternative physician.

The American Holistic Medical Association is a reputable organization of holistic physicians. While it can't certify the standards of its members, many doctors who belong to this group are excellent. The address is 4101 Lake Boone Trail #201, Raleigh, NC 26707. The phone number is (919) 787- 5146.

Working with Doctors of Osteopathy (D.O.s)

Osteopathic physicians today possess a license that is legally equivalent to that of M.D.s. They function in all of the categories of medicine, from family practice to neurosurgery. However, the history of osteopathy has left a legacy of greater openness to alternative approaches. Osteopathic medicine started out as an alternative approach itself, focusing on manual manipulation and natural therapies, and some medical students today choose schools of osteopathy because they are particularly interested in alternative medicine. For this reason, some D.O.s may be more open to St. John's wort than the average M.D.

It isn't always the case, however. The majority of osteopaths function identically to M.D.s, and many have expanded beyond conventional medical practice only so far as to include manual manipulative techniques. For these physicians, you will need to use the approaches described in the preceding section.

Other Alternative Practitioners

There are several categories of health care providers that focus primarily on alternative health care techniques. While their interest in herbs such as St. John's wort can be taken as a given, their knowledge of the medical side of the equation may not always be adequate.

Naturopathic Physicians

One of the most promising categories of alternative practitioners is doctors of naturopathy, or N.D.s. These physicians specialize in treatments such as herbs, vitamins, and food supplements. Their education is quite good, consisting of four years of postgraduate training at an accredited naturopathic college. In school, naturopathic physicians receive considerable education in conventional diagnosis and treatment, along with alternative approaches. This gives them a good balance, except that their practical, hands-on training is far less than that of M.D.s or D.O.s.

Nonetheless, naturopaths are typically responsible, levelheaded practitioners. It is unfortunate that only a handful of states recognize the N.D. degree.

All naturopaths are familiar with the use of St. John's wort. Indeed, the naturopath Michael Murray was one of the first to popularize standardized St. John's wort extract in the United States. Nevertheless, their relative lack of clinical experience with acute illnesses may make naturopaths significantly less skillful than D.O.s and M.D.s at recognizing the warning signs of severe major depression. This limits the usefulness of naturopathic consultation for those considering the use of St. John's wort.

Doctors of Chiropractic

In many states, chiropractors are permitted to prescribe herbs and food supplements. Their education typically covers much of the same ground that is covered in naturopathic school, although there is a greater emphasis on spinal manipulation, of course. Most chiropractors have studied herbal medicine, at least to some extent, although the scientific side of herbology seems to be stressed less in chiropractic school than in naturopathic training. Some chiropractors may seek additional education to supplement their knowledge.

Unfortunately, just like naturopathic physicians, chiropractors may be insufficiently experienced in the signs of severe major depression to notice the early warning signals.

Nutritionists

Numerous individuals call themselves nutritionists, but the term does not indicate any universally accepted standard of education. Nutritionists typically recommend herbs and food supplements. Unfortunately, their sophistication in doing so is highly variable. Many have not studied the scientific side of herbal medicine, and few possess adequate training in psychological conditions such as depression.

Psychologists and Psychotherapists

Unlike psychiatrists, psychologists and psychotherapists are not medical doctors. Nevertheless, they are usually very well versed in the ins and outs of depression. Most can recognize the signs of severe major depression more readily than a typical primary care physician.

Because St. John's wort is sold as a food supplement and not a drug, there is nothing to stop psychologists and psychotherapists from recommending it to their clients. (Technically, this may be practicing medicine without a license, but in real life there is no serious obstacle.) An increasing number of these health care professionals have begun to delve into this and other natural approaches to the treatment of emotional illnesses. In many cases, they provide a high level of expertise.

CHAPTER TEN

Other Alternative Treatments for Depression

• Ginkgo biloba	• Lifestyle changes
• DL-phenylalanine	• Supplemental treatments for anxiety
• Phosphatidyl serine	
• Nutrient deficiencies	• Supplemental treatments for insomnia
• Food allergies	

Alternative medicine is an immense field, almost a world unto itself. While some approaches within this world are ridiculous, others are reasonably practical, and a few are fully as scientific as most conventional treatments. This complex subject is discussed more fully in my book *The Alternative Medicine Sourcebook: A Realistic Evaluation of Alternative Healing Options* (Lowell House, 1997).

None of the techniques described in this chapter have been as solidly researched as St. John's wort. However, most have some research backing, and all seem to work at least occasionally. Alternative practitioners frequently combine these methods with St. John's wort to augment its effect. They can also be used as a substitute for St. John's wort when the herb fails to produce satisfactory results.

Ginkgo Biloba

The ginkgo biloba tree is a beautiful ornamental that can grow more than 100 feet tall and live for longer than 1,000 years. It has been called "the living fossil" because evidence of its existence can be traced back more than 200 million years. Once distributed on many continents, it was nearly wiped out during the Ice Ages and survived only in China. However, the resilience it developed during its long tenure on earth has given it the power to survive a new hostile environment: that of modern city streets. Because of its superb resistance to insects, disease, and air pollution, ginkgo has become a widely planted sidewalk decoration.

The medicinal use of ginkgo goes back to ancient China, where its leaves were used as a standard part of the extensive Chinese medical repertoire. Its traditional uses included "benefiting the brain" as well as aiding respiratory illnesses and ridding the body of parasitic worms.

In modern times, standardized extracts of the ginkgo leaf have been extensively researched in Europe. Most of the research into ginkgo has concentrated on its ability to improve circulation in the brain and extremities. Favorable results in over forty double-blind studies have led to its widespread European use for impaired mental function due to insufficient blood flow to the brain (cerebral vascular insufficiency). Ginkgo is also prescribed for intermittent claudication, the pain with exercise that occurs when arteries are blocked by atherosclerotic changes. According to the respected naturopath Michael Murray, ginkgo extract accounts for 1.5 percent of all prescription sales in France and 1 percent of those in Germany.[56]

During the studies on impaired mental functions, researchers frequently observed improvements in mood and relief from symptoms of depression. This incidental discovery led scientists to investigate whether ginkgo might be useful as an antidepressant treatment. One study published in 1990 evaluated this effect in sixty inpatients with depressive symptoms.[57] The results showed significant improvements among patients given ginkgo extract instead of placebo.

Another study followed forty depressed patients over the age of fifty who had not responded successfully to antidepressant treatment.[58] Those who were given ginkgo showed an average drop in HAM-D scores of 50 percent, while the placebo group showed only a 10 percent improvement.

In 1994 an interesting piece of research was reported that may shed light on the mechanism by which ginkgo improves depression.[59] This study examined levels of serotonin receptors in rats of various ages. When older rats were given ginkgo, the level of serotonin binding sites increased. The same effect was *not* observed, however, in younger rats. The researchers theorized that ginkgo may block an age-related loss of serotonin receptors.

Reduced receptors for serotonin may mean that the body needs more serotonin to produce a normal effect. Instead of raising the level of serotonin, like Prozac, ginkgo may thus improve the brain's ability to respond to serotonin (at least in older people). But this is still highly speculative. More experimentation is needed to both clarify the mechanism of ginkgo's action and better quantify its effectiveness in depression.

Nonetheless, the clinical results of ginkgo are strong enough that it is already widely used for depression. Scott Shannon ordinarily combines ginkgo with St. John's wort when treating depression in patients over fifty. Many commercial St. John's wort products include ginkgo in appropriate doses.

In my own practice, I've seen many patients who reported significant improvement through taking ginkgo extract. One of the most dramatic cases is Marilyn, a woman who in her late sixties had become morose and withdrawn. Fearing Alzheimer's disease, her daughter had given Marilyn ginkgo, hoping it would improve her mental functioning. The results were dramatic. In about three weeks, Marilyn was back to macramé, letter writing, and going for long walks with her friends.

She continued this way for a year. Then, due to the expense, Marilyn stopped taking ginkgo. Within a month she was living in her recliner again.

A subsequent medical evaluation showed that Marilyn didn't have Alzheimer's. She was merely depressed. Her physician then prescribed Prozac, with excellent results. However, ginkgo had worked just as well. In this case, the natural treatment was just as effective as the drug.

Of course, ginkgo doesn't always work, but there is no known risk involved in trying it. Among 9,722 patients who were given the herb in double-blind studies, the most common side effect was mild stomach discomfort; and it only occurred in about 0.2 percent of the studied patients.[60] Headaches and dizziness were the next most common problems.

Although side effects are nearly nonexistent, ginkgo is expensive, ranging from $20 to $50 dollars per month. The proper dose is 40 to 80 milligrams three times daily of an extract standardized to contain 24 percent ginkgo flavonoid glycosides (heterosides). It may take two to eight weeks for the full antidepressant effect to develop.

Phenylalanine (DLPA)

Phenylalanine is a naturally occurring amino acid that we all consume in our daily diets. Artificial supplementation with phenylalanine seems sometimes to be effective in the treatment of depression. Many alternative practitioners use it along with St. John's wort and report enhanced results.

The body can convert phenylalanine into a variety of biological amines. While this may eventually explain its antidepressant benefits, what is known thus far about its mechanism of action can only be regarded as highly preliminary and speculative. That it is effective for depression is somewhat better documented.

Phenylalanine occurs in a right-hand and a left-hand form, known as D- and L-phenylalanine respectively. Some studies have evaluated the D form, and others the L form, while still others evaluated mixtures of both. The mixed DL form (DLPA) is the product most commonly available in stores.

A 1978 study compared the effectiveness of D-phenylalanine against the antidepressant drug imipramine, given in the somewhat low (but probably effective) dose of 100 milligrams daily.[61] A total of sixty patients were randomly assigned to either one group or the other and followed for thirty days. The results in both groups were statistically equivalent. However, D-phenylalanine worked more rapidly, producing significant improvement in only fifteen days.

Another double-blind study followed twenty-seven patients, half of whom received DL-phenylalanine and the other half imipramine in full doses of 150 to 200 milligrams.[62] When they were reevaluated in thirty days, the two groups had improved by the same statistical margin.

Unfortunately, I have been unable to find any good studies that directly compared phenylalanine to placebo. Several such studies have been performed, but they were all too small or too flawed to be worth reporting. Nonetheless, phenylalanine seems to be effective in practice. I recently surveyed a panel of expert alternative practitioners in order to provide the data for another book on which I am working. DL-phenylalanine was one of the most popular antidepressant treatments, rated at a level of "often effective."

I have known numerous patients to benefit from DLPA. One such was a thirty-two-year-old salesman named Randy, who had found himself increasingly unmotivated at work. He enjoyed his job and was successful at it, but he was finding it increasingly difficult to keep his focus. "It's not like me," he would say. "I feel so gloomy when I get to work."

I suggested that he might be subconsciously interested in changing his career, but he adamantly opposed that theory. "The job's great," he said. "The people are great, I believe in my product, and the money's good. This depression is coming out of nowhere."

Because I wouldn't stop suggesting psychological angles, Randy finally quit seeing me, and visited a naturopath instead. I didn't hear from him for three months. Then he called to let me know what had worked, and even before he told me anything about the treatment I was already impressed by how good he sounded.

"I started taking DL-phenylalanine about a month ago. The stuff's incredible. I don't even remember what it feels like to be depressed."

His voice was sparkling and full of life. When I asked him what he had tried the first two months, he said, "First she put me on some kind of wort. John's wort, or something like that. It didn't do a thing. But this DL-phenylalanine, it's powerful."

Of course, this amino acid doesn't always succeed, either. If St. John's wort helps about 50 to 75 percent of those with mild to moderate depression, DL-phenylalanine alone is probably only effective in 25 to 50 percent of those who take it. Fortunately, it isn't always the same people for whom they both work. If one treatment fails, the other may be worth a try; and they can also be combined for an augmented effect.

In clinical practice, most physicians prescribe from 150 to 400 milligrams daily of DL-phenylalanine, divided up into two or three daily doses. Side effects are rare, although increased anxiety, headache, and even mild hypertension have been occasionally reported when higher doses of phenylalanine were used. Phenylalanine must be avoided by those with the rare metabolic disease phenylketonuria (PKU). Because of the risk that a child may have undiagnosed PKU, some authorities recommend that pregnant and nursing women shouldn't take phenylalanine.

The related amino acid tyrosine is sometimes mentioned as a proven treatment for depression, but in actual fact the few published studies are so poor they aren't worth mentioning. Nonetheless, tyrosine supplementation is sometimes helpful. The proper dose seems to fall in the neighborhood of 300 milligrams three times a day, and there are no side effects.

Phosphatidyl Serine

Phosphatidyl serine is one of the chemicals that the body uses to maintain the integrity of cell membranes, and it is the primary such chemical used in the brain.[63] It is not an essential nutrient because cells can manufacture this substance themselves. However, when taken as a food supplement phosphatidyl serine sometimes seems to improve brain function.

Most of the research on this chemical has concentrated on elderly patients with mental impairment. One double-blind study followed 494 patients with Alzheimer's-like symptoms for six months, and the results demonstrated that phosphatidyl serine improved mental function, mood, and behavior.[64] So far only one study has concentrated on this substance's effectiveness in depression.[65] The results appear to be favorable, but further research needs to be done.

In clinical practice, physicians who use phosphatidyl serine report marked improvement in some depressed patients over fifty. It seems to be most beneficial in patients for whom mental decline is an important part of the picture.

As an example, I once prescribed phosphatidyl serine to a husband and wife, both of whom were in their sixties and suffering from depression. The reason I used this supplement instead of St. John's wort was that the husband suffered from an Alzheimer's-like syndrome. I had hoped that phosphatidyl serine might improve his mental abilities, and the wife had requested that they both be able to take the same pill.

The results were excellent. The wife's depression abated first, but the husband's state of mind soon improved as well; and his cognitive abilities also increased noticeably. At the time of this writing, six years later, they are still taking phosphatidyl serine and doing well.

The proper dose of phosphatidyl serine is 100 milligrams three times daily. Full results take anywhere from four weeks to six months to manifest. Although there do not seem to be any side effects, this is a very expensive supplement, usually costing in the range of $50 to $75 per month. Another drawback is that phosphatidyl serine isn't really a natural medicine. It's produced semisynthetically from soy lecithin.

Nutrient Deficiencies

Contrary to what you might read, treatment with phenylalanine or phosphatidyl serine should not really be considered nutritional medicine. Most Americans receive satisfactory amounts of phenylalanine in their daily diet, and phosphatidyl serine is not normally consumed orally at all.

A true nutritional treatment corrects a dietary deficiency. Depression can be a symptom of inadequate intake of folic acid, vitamin B_6, vitamin B_{12}, magnesium, iron, and essential fatty acids. Since studies have shown widespread deficiencies in these common nutrients,[66] it is reasonable to assume that in some cases of depression simple supplementation may make a difference.

Except for the fatty acids, these nutrients can be easily supplemented through standard vitamin and mineral pills. The best source of "good" essential fatty acids is probably cold-water fish, but a reasonable substitute is the supplement flax oil, taken at a dose of one or two tablespoons a day.

Despite the logic behind such supplementation, in actual clinical practice I have rarely heard of anyone who's depression was cured simply by taking a multivitamin. It seems that while severe deficiency of common nutrients can certainly cause depression, slight deficiencies rarely produce noticeable effects. Supplementation may still be helpful as a supportive treatment.

Food Allergies

While the alternative treatments for depression suggested thus far are simple to implement, since they consist merely of taking pills, food allergy treatment is a much more complex approach. For many people, it is too arduous and can even lead to a kind of obsession with food, for which I've coined the tongue-in-cheek term *orthorexia nervosa* (fixation on eating the right food).[67] Nonetheless, it is sometimes quite effective.

Food allergies come in two varieties: the immediate, severe form that involves hives or even bee-sting-like anaphylactic reactions, and the more common, delayed form that causes a wide variety of subtle symptoms. It is the second type that can cause depression.

Milk allergy is probably the most common example of the delayed-onset type. After drinking milk regularly for a period of days to several weeks, those who are allergic to it typically experience increased mucus, asthma, eczema, fatigue, or frequent colds. Other symptoms of delayed food allergies may include depression, joint pain, sinus infection, headache, digestive disturbance, impairment of concentration, bloating, fluid retention, and, indeed, practically any other symptom you can name.

In order of prevalence, the most common food allergens are milk, wheat, corn, soy, and eggs. Some people also develop allergiclike reactions to sugar, caffeine, and alcohol, although a classic, actual allergic response is not occurring. In order to take this type of reaction into account, it may be preferable to use the term "food sensitivities" or "trigger foods" instead of "food allergies."

Conventional medicine prefers to focus on dramatic and obvious conditions, in order to avoid the fuzzy realm of subjective experience. For this reason, it recognizes primarily the first type of food allergy and leaves the entire subject of delayed food sensitivities to practitioners of alternative medicine. Food allergies are a major concern of naturopaths, nutritionists, and many alternative M.D.s.

Diagnosing Delayed Food Allergies

It isn't always easy to sort out which foods are causing health problems, because the effects are delayed and prolonged and many foods may be involved. The only absolutely effective diagnostic technique is the elimination diet followed by food challenges. In this method, you eat a fantastically simplified diet for about a month, or until your chronic symptoms begin to "clear." This usually consists solely of turkey, lamb, yams, and white rice.

Next, you introduce foods at the rate of about one a week. Those that cause definite reactions in a day or so are identified as strong allergens that may need to be avoided forever. Those that cause symptoms only after being eaten for several days in a row, however, may be acceptable when eaten occasionally on a "rotation" schedule. Other foods may prove to be entirely harmless and can be eaten at will. (Yams, white rice, lamb, and turkey fall into this category for almost everyone, which is why they may be eaten during the elimination phase.)

The food-elimination–food-challenge method takes considerable courage, willpower, and self-denial. Since not everyone is up to such an ascetic practice, alternative practitioners have expended a great deal of effort trying to come up with laboratory tests that can provide the same information. Skin tests have been proven highly unreliable. But blood tests that examine the blood for antibodies against foods have a somewhat better track record, and they can provide a rough indication of what foods to avoid. One caution, though: the lab report must always be matched against actual experience.

Benefits and Side Effects of Trigger-Food Avoidance

There are no good research studies on the subject, but in clinical practice cutting down on trigger foods can sometimes provide dramatic relief from depression. I remember one patient whose painful history of recurrent depression proved to be primarily due to excessive caffeine consumption, and the case of another patient, Mary-Ann, was even more dramatic. After years of treatment for severe major depression, during which time Mary-Ann had been hospitalized twice and treated with six different antidepressants, a naturopath suggested she quit eating wheat. The results were so powerful that within three months she was off all medication and felt better than she had in many years.

Food allergen identification and avoidance is a rather hit-and-miss treatment, however. While it sometimes produces good results—even in severe illnesses—it very often does nothing at all. I regard this method as a difficult approach with a relatively low success rate.

Furthermore, even when it is successful, trigger-food avoidance often produces severe "side effects." Patients who try to eat very carefully frequently end up with a restricted social life and a preoccupation with diet. Over time, an increasing number of foods may gradually begin to cause problems, until the sufferer can eat practically nothing at all with impunity. The numerous side effects of Prozac may pale in comparison to the results of food allergen fanaticism.

For this reason, I seldom recommend trigger-food avoidance except when it is limited to a few fairly simple foods, or to nonfoods, such as caffeine and alcohol. Almost any alternative may be worth trying instead.

Lifestyle Changes

Thus far, this chapter has primarily focused on treatment options for depression that consist of specific, targeted methods. These approaches are the easiest to use and evaluate, but by concentrating on them, I've invited fierce criticism from my colleagues in alternative medicine. "We're supposed to treat the whole person," they say to me, and I have to agree.

The best approach to any illness is a holistic one that involves many dimensions of the self. I've previously stressed the importance of psychotherapy, but it may also be essential to consider the impact of lifestyle factors. In the clinic, I always ask questions such as: Do you exercise? What's your stress level? Do you have a good diet? And do you enjoy your job, your social life, and your living situation?

If you don't take care of yourself as a whole person, it's quite possible that more specific treatments will fail to work. Probably the simplest lifestyle intervention is to increase your exercise level. Numerous clinical studies seem to indicate that exercise is an effective antidepressant. While other studies contradict this intuitive result, the least that can be said is that it won't hurt. Exercise increases overall health and energy, reduces the risk of many illnesses, and relieves stress.

Speaking of stress, there is no question that excessive stress can put most anyone into a depression. Although life is inevitably full of stresses, there are numerous activities that can moderate their impact. Some of the most useful include regular exercise, meditation, prayer, good social interactions, play, visualizations, regular massage, and an extended vacation.

It is also important to consider the effects of overall diet. Psychoactive substances such as caffeine, alcohol, and even chocolate may lead to increased depression in many people. Other substances, such as sugar and fat, can increase depression in a few. As previously mentioned, dietary deficiencies of important nutrients may sometimes play a role in depression as well. Good diet, like regular exercise, provides numerous health benefits, so it certainly fits into the "couldn't hurt" category.

Finally, depression can be caused by life choices and situations. If you are in an abusive marriage, if you hate your job, or if you have no friends, depression is the likely result. An excessive focus on status and money and not enough on love can also make you miserable. This last subject is the topic of innumerable plays, movies, and books—not to mention religious scripture—and it has never stopped being true.

I remember a man in his forties who came to me when Prozac failed to alleviate his depression. His was a life devoted solely to the pursuit of progressively higher standing in the state bureaucracy of Washington. My first impression was that he was miserable because his priorities were confused. Never did he spend more than two hours a week with his children, although he bought them expensive presents, and his primary idea of a good time seemed to be buttering up superiors and scheming against competitors. For recreation, he watched the news and ate hamburgers.

I couldn't imagine anyone being happy living the way he did and told him so. However, he couldn't understand what I was talking about and reacted angrily. "I want an herb," he said, "not a bunch of moralizing."

Intimidated, I prescribed him St. John's wort, but it didn't do him any good. He didn't actually change until he suffered a heart attack two years later. This catastrophe opened his eyes, and he actually began to institute major changes in his life. Fortunately, his heart wasn't badly damaged, and he has a good chance of living a more satisfying life for many years.

Changing deeply embedded life patterns can be quite difficult. Nevertheless, there are ways to accomplish it without nearly dying. Friends, counselors, clergy, social workers, and physicians all may be able to assist you in initiating positive changes. Sometimes the boost of an antidepressant (whether herbal or pharmaceutical) may also be useful as a kind of "jump-start."

Supplemental Treatments for Anxiety

Anxiety frequently accompanies depression. While relief from anxiety symptoms may result from taking St. John's wort, it may only be after the herb's full effect develops in four to six weeks. Sometimes a more rapidly acting treatment is needed. Conventional medicine uses a group of drugs called anxiolytics for this purpose. Unfortunately, most of them are habit-forming—sometimes severely so—and they all can cause decreases in mental function. Alternative medicine has at least a couple of good options that can be tried instead.

The most scientifically validated herbal treatment for anxiety is the root of the Piper methysticum plant, commonly known as kava. This member of the pepper family has long been cultivated by Pacific Islanders. They make a drink out of kava and consume it on ceremonial occasions. In small doses, this drink produces relaxation, while larger doses induce sleep.

Standardized extracts of kava have been approved in Europe for the treatment of anxiety and insomnia, and it is used widely for those purposes. Several double-blind studies document kava's effectiveness. For example, one study published in 1991 followed fifty-eight patients with anxiety, half of whom received kava extract and the other half placebo.[68] Over the course of four weeks the Hamilton Anxiety Scale (analogous to the HAM-D scale used for depression) was administered to rate the level of anxiety. The HAM-A quantifies symptoms such as restlessness, nervousness, heart palpitations, stomach discomfort, dizziness, and chest pain. Patients given kava instead of placebo showed dramatically better results than those on placebo, without significant side effects.

Other studies have compared kava against oxazepam, a conventional anxiolytic. One of these comparisons demonstrated that while oxazepam and similar drugs impair alertness, kava may actually improve some measures of mental performance.[69]

In private practice, I've sometimes seen kava produce dramatic results. For example, one patient complained of depression, anxiety, and panic attacks that developed suddenly after she graduated from college. It seemed that the stress produced by facing "the real world" was temporarily overpowering her. Since she strongly preferred herbal treatment to medication, I started her on St. John's wort.

When its benefits didn't occur rapidly enough, she returned to my office requesting additional assistance. I started her on kava preparation, and within a week she said she felt substantially better. Eventually she quit taking the St. John's wort altogether because it bothered her stomach and used kava alone periodically for about a year. At the end of that time she had found a career and no longer needed any form of treatment.

Despite this impressive success story, in clinical practice kava is usually not as potent as drugs. Its lack of side effects, however, may make it worth trying first. The standard dose is 100 milligrams, three times a day, of an extract standardized to contain 70 percent kavalactones.

However, this typical preparation of kava may not be the optimum form. Kavalactones don't seem to be the only ingredient essential to the treatment of anxiety. Just as with St. John's wort, where hypericin is not the only factor, the "minor" ingredients of kava may be needed to produce its anti-anxiety effect. In support of this theory, 100 percent kavalactone preparations generally prove to be *less* effective than the 70 percent extract. According to some authorities, a 30 percent concentration is the ideal, because it includes higher concentrations of unrecognized but still important constituents.

Kava's anti-anxiety effects usually begin within a week and continue to increase over an additional two weeks. At standard doses, kava does not generally cause any side effects. A few reports indicate that it may worsen symptoms of Parkinson's disease, however, so it is not recommended for those with that illness. Ten times the normal dose can cause a particular skin eruption known as kava dermopathy. One hundred times the standard dose may cause a variety of changes on lab tests, although those patients in whom this effect has been observed were also alcoholics, making any conclusions suspect.[70]

Besides kava, there are also a number of European herbs traditionally used for anxiety, including hops, lady's slipper, skullcap, lobelia, and rauwolfia. However, the effects of these other herbs seem to be rather mild and yet at the same time may present real dangers if used in excessive doses.

Other useful treatments for anxiety include calcium (1,000 milligrams a day), magnesium (500 milligrams a day), and vitamin B_6 (50 milligrams a day). These food supplements may be particularly effective in the anxiety associated with PMS. Acupuncture is also sometimes effective for anxiety.

Supplemental Treatments for Insomnia

Insomnia is another symptom that commonly goes along with depression. Just as for anxiety, there are a number of alternative treatments that may be useful while waiting for St. John's wort to kick in.

Probably the most proven alternative treatment for insomnia is the herb valerian. Small double-blind studies have shown that valerian is significantly more effective than placebo, without producing morning sleepiness.[71] Valerian's benefits for insomnia occur without the side effects of morning sleepiness, daytime drowsiness, or disturbances of sleep stages.

In clinical practice, valerian is useful but seldom as powerful as pharmaceutical sleeping pills. It is best described as a mild sedative, and, unfortunately, its benefits usually wear off with extended use.

The proper dose of valerian is 1 to 2 grams of dried root, or 150 to 300 milligrams of valerian extract standardized to 0.8 percent valeric acid. It should be taken twenty minutes before bedtime. While valerian is generally regarded as safe, it has a highly unpleasant odor.

Kava is another option for insomnia, taken at a dose of 200 to 300 milligrams one hour before bed. Other herbs used for insomnia include hops, passionflower, lady's slipper, skullcap, and lobelia. These herbs are generally less effective than kava or valerian, however, and some can be dangerous if taken to excess.

Acupuncture is occasionally dramatically effective for insomnia. Although there are no good studies to prove it, clinically speaking there are some people who achieve dramatic, lasting results from six to ten acupuncture sessions. But this is a relatively expensive form of treatment, and one whose overall success rate is less than stunning.

Finally, visualization tapes, meditation, and yoga may make falling asleep easier and even improve sleep quality.

CHAPTER ELEVEN

Future Directions

- Improved research
- New routes through the FDA approval process
- Overcoming bias on both sides
- If St. John's wort were approved as a drug
- Other treatments on the way
- What this means for the future of alternative medicine

With St. John's wort, herbal medicine may be on the verge of a breakthrough. Never before has an herb achieved such widespread recognition and respect based on good scientific evidence. Yet there still remain many obstacles to overcome before the conventional medical establishment can accept this traditional treatment. This chapter proposes what steps should be taken next and envisions what St. John's wort may bring to the future of conventional and alternative medicine.

Improved Research

No herb has ever been licensed as a medical treatment in this country. For this reason, it will be necessary to achieve particularly high standards of research to leap the hurdle of settled history. The published scientific studies of St. John's wort, while impressive, still fall short in certain essential respects.

Some of the charges leveled against the published St. John's wort trials can be dismissed out of hand. For example, complaints that the studies lasted only five to six weeks can be disregarded because that is the standard length of drug trials prior to approval. Criticism that St. John's wort was not evaluated for severe major depression is similarly inappropriate, since no one is proposing it as a treatment for severe major depression. There are, however, several real problems in the research record that do need to be addressed:

- No studies were performed in the United States.
- Many studies used outdated classification systems for depression.
- The physicians performing the HAM-D test did not undertake joint training to minimize variation in how they interpreted results.
- Comparisons against pharmaceutical treatments did not use therapeutic levels of the comparison drugs.

With some effort, each of these legitimate criticisms can be overcome.

Conducting U.S. Trials

Considering the intense publicity now surrounding St. John's wort, it shouldn't be difficult to recruit researchers interested in performing studies. The only real obstacle is obtaining funding. Drug companies are the source of most medical research dollars, but they can't be expected to fund research into St. John's wort extracts because they do not manufacture it.

Rather, the appropriate source of funds would be those companies who already sell St. John's wort. Alternative medicine has long complained that no one funds research into alternative methods; it may now be time to take responsibility instead of complaining. After all, pharmaceutical companies didn't get any handouts when *they* were getting started. I suggest that a consortium of St. John's wort manufacturers pool their funds and institute serious, independent research into the effectiveness of the product they sell.

If the studies are properly performed, they will doubtless provide positive results, and the outcome will be increased sales and heightened prestige for the manufacturers. The credibility of other products manufactured by the same companies will also rise, leading to greater income and the possibility of additional research. (The problem of patentability is discussed later in this chapter.)

Using Modern Classification Systems for Depression

Only the Hansgen study (described in chapter 5) used the most up-to-date definition of depression, drawn from the *DSM III*. All other studies used outdated diagnostic systems (ICD-9) and old-fashioned terms, such as "neurotic depression" and "psycho-vegetative symptoms." This could easily be remedied in U.S. trials. Patients could be selected on the basis of the *DSM* definition of dysthymia or major depression and classified as to severity by using the HAM-D rating scale.

Joint Training of Physicians

When rating scales such as the HAM-D are used, the most reliable results can be obtained through training the examining physicians in the same classroom and then testing them to see if they come up with similar evaluations of given patients. The technical description for this procedure is "assuring interoperator reliability." While not all studies of antidepressant drugs employ this method, the best ones do; and it raises the prestige of the results. U.S. trials of St. John's wort should follow suit.

Improving Comparisons with Chemical Antidepressants

As described in chapter 7, all the published studies that compared St. John's wort to drug treatment were essentially invalid because they used too low a dose of the comparator drug. The net result is studies that give the impression of being intentionally deceptive.

Actually, the German researchers who performed comparison trials used low doses of drugs on purpose. They knew that drugs cause side effects, and they wanted to keep the double-blind setup intact. If patients had been given full doses of drugs, they would have been able to guess by their dry mouths and sleepiness that they were in the drug, rather than the herb, subgroup, which could trigger the placebo effect.

But lowering the dose of the drug is not a good solution to the problem. A better way might be to compare full doses of gold-standard antidepressants (such as imipramine) against a combination of St. John's wort and an antihistamine. Imipramine's side effects are identical to those of Benedryl, and since no one believes that Benedryl is an antidepressant in itself, such a comparison would preserve the double-blind and provide meaningful results.

For comparisons between St. John's wort and Prozac, perhaps both treatments could be combined with small amounts of caffeine. This would tend to equalize the stimulant effects, balance the influence of suggestion, and thus eliminate unequal distribution of the placebo effect. (The reason to combine caffeine with *both* substances is that caffeine itself can occasionally cause depression, so it should be administered to both groups. Too, caffeine's stimulant effects are more overt than those of Prozac.)

Such studies should also include polling to determine whether patients and physicians could guess which treatment was which. If the results showed a guessing rate better than 50 percent, it would mean that the double-blind wasn't being maintained. (The same type of polling should be required for drug studies as well!) If this polling showed that patients and physicians were remaining in the dark, the validity of the results would be substantiated.

However, there still remains the hurdle of the FDA.

New Routes Through the FDA Approval Process

For St. John's wort to become the first herb to be approved as a drug, it would have to pass through the FDA's certification process. This process is presently so expensive and arduous that, unless it is changed, no nonpatentable substance will ever be able to make it through. The following advocates changing the FDA's rules to facilitate the approval of unpatentables.

The drug approval process as it is presently constituted involves three major phases, beginning with animal studies. As previously mentioned, there is a good reason for the complexity of this process: to prevent disasters. If thorough animal studies had been required in the '50s, for example, thalidomide would never have been released.

Many of the FDA's precautionary methods simply don't make sense, however, for substances already in wide use. No one had taken thalidomide until it was invented. But millions of people have taken St. John's wort in Germany, and at least many thousands have taken it in the United States. There is really no need now to step cautiously through animal studies and small-dose human studies. St. John's wort can ethically be given at full doses in clinical trials right now because so many people are already taking it at full doses!

In the European community there are streamlined procedures in place to simplify the approval process for substances already known to be safe. A similarly sensible shortcut should be adopted here.

But one more step is necessary. Those who risk the money on researching unpatentable substances need a certain level of protection. Otherwise, there is nothing to stop outside companies from cashing in once FDA approval is achieved.

There is precedent for giving special status to a class of substances in order to facilitate their approval and distribution: the Orphan Drug Act. This law, enacted in 1983, gives favorable treatment to medications for rare or unusual diseases. Without such help, drug companies would not market such drugs, because the limited market would prevent them from making enough money through sales to pay back the costs of research. Direct grants, loans, special patent provisions, and other incentives help overcome this economic obstacle.

Similarly, unpatentable substances deserve special legislation. It makes no scientific sense that unpatentables should be kept from approval for purely financial reasons. After all, there is no reason to believe that a substance may not be effective simply because it escapes patent laws. Indeed, it seems logical to suspect that certain unpatentable substances, such as vitamins and other food supplements, might be safer on average than new drugs.

Perhaps all the manufacturers who would collectively pay for research into such a substance could be granted a special kind of patent, allowing them the right to market that substance exclusively for a certain period of years. Alternatively, a fund could be established that would pay back the costs of research through a tax on future sales of the substance, no matter who sold it, to be discontinued once the initial expenses were defrayed. Other incentives might also be necessary to facilitate such useful but potentially unprofitable research.

Nevertheless, there is still one more major obstacle to overcome.

Overcoming Bias on Both Sides

No doubt the FDA and the conventional medical establishment would resist any attempt to license herbs as drugs. Vitamins and other nutritional chemicals are already the subject of widespread scientific study and enthusiastic discussion in medical journals, but herbs are a different subject.

Physicians have no problem calling vitamin E a drug and studying its effectiveness in various diseases, because it is a single, isolated substance. However, as I described in chapter 9, herbs make scientists uncomfortable because they are complex mixtures of thousands of naturally occurring chemicals. Utilizing a whole herb instead of an active ingredient manufactured from that herb seems to a medical researcher an unreliable and unreproducible technique that is distasteful to the scientific ethic.

Thus, attempts to legitimize herbal medicine encounter resistance. The FDA seems to bend over backwards to approve drugs, even if the proof of efficacy is weak (as Peter Breggin points out so convincingly in *Talking Back to Prozac*); but it would undoubtedly throw up numerous obstacles to approving any herb, no matter how well it was researched. Only public pressure can overcome this bias.

But there is an equal level of bias on the other side. Most alternative practitioners are suspicious of the FDA, to put it mildly. For decades, alternative practitioners have attacked the FDA and pharmaceutical companies as part of a conspiracy to suppress safe, natural treatments. Such a history can't be set aside easily. Going through the necessary process to obtain approval for St. John's wort would seem to many involved in alternative medicine like "dealing with the devil." They would enter the process suspicious, combative, and expecting a trap.

And the supplement industry isn't likely to jump at the chance to pay for high-quality research into alternative treatments. After all, this multibillion-dollar industry has never even agreed to a uniform standard for quality control. Although it has long complained of not being treated with respect, it has also benefited economically by its lax standards. Taking on the responsibility for funding thorough, independent research at respectable institutions would present a new challenge that many supplement companies would resist.

Nonetheless, this problem of mutual bias can be solved. The FDA can be encouraged to overcome its objections to multi-ingredient herbal medicines by pointing out that some drugs already in use contain numerous ingredients. "Conjugated estrogens," for example, are a mixture of different hormones commonly prescribed to postmenopausal women. And reputable researchers have recently described the "mixed tocopherol" form of vitamin E as superior to the pure "alpha tocopherol" form. Given these precedents, a whole herbal extract such as St. John's wort should also be potentially acceptable.

On the alternative medicine side of the conflict, it will be necessary for advocates to change their point of view from "permanent outsider" to "potential insider." There is precedent for this too. Just as many of the 1960s generation finally decided to work within the system to change it instead of vilifying it from without, alternative medicine can take that same step and embrace the potentialities and responsibilities of mainstream acceptance.

If St. John's Wort Were Approved As a Drug

If the many obstacles described above can be overcome, St. John's wort might very well be the first herb to achieve approved status. The consequence would be that medical physicians would become much more likely to prescribe it, and many more patients would be thus encouraged to try it. Millions would benefit who presently endure the side effects of prescription drugs, or who endure mild to moderate depression because they can't tolerate those side effects.

Under FDA scrutiny, St. John's wort preparations would become more standardized and reliable, and the nagging question of product quality would fade away. Furthermore, success with this herb would accustom both physicians and patients to accepting herbal treatments in general. This would help bring the ethic of "sticking closer to nature" back into the conventional medical world.

Such a change has already begun. It was not very many decades ago that medical physicians recommended baby formula over nursing, because it was "more scientific." Doctors also paid next to no attention to diet and nutrition, allowing many hospital patients to essentially starve on IV glucose drips and ignoring the benefits of a healthful diet as disease prevention. But now, even the most conservative medical institutions devote considerable attention to nutrition.

I was recently amused to hear a radio interview at the Sloan Kettering Cancer Institute, wherein the spokesperson recommended a high-fiber, high-fruit and -vegetable, low-fat diet for preventing cancer. "Diet is the most exciting new frontier of cancer research," he said in conclusion; and I nearly rear-ended the car in front of me when I heard it.

Approval of St. John's wort would facilitate the progression of this process. The culture of conventional medicine would open just a bit wider, and physicians would soon be encouraged to look in more friendly fashion on numerous approaches that are presently "alternative."

Other Treatments on the Way

Several vitamins and food supplements are already on a fast track toward acceptance. Vitamin E is routinely referred to in medical literature as a drug; and other antioxidants, such as vitamin C and carotene, are presently undergoing intensive study. Other reasonable candidates for approved drug status based on their research record include glucosamine sulfate (osteoarthritis), coenzyme Q_{10} (hypertension, congestive heart failure, and cardiomyopathy), aortic glycosaminoglycans (varicose veins and hemorrhoids), phosphatidyl choline (liver disorders, high cholesterol), carnitine (various cardiovascular diseases), phosphatidyl serine (cognitive impairment in the elderly), and omega-3 fatty acids (cardiovascular disease, rheumatoid arthritis).

Besides these chemical food supplements, a number of standardized herbal extracts are also good candidates for approval: feverfew (migraines), garlic (high cholesterol and other cardiovascular risk factors), ginkgo (cerebral and peripheral vascular insufficiency), goldenseal (topical antibiotic), saw palmetto (benign prostatic hypertrophy), hawthorne (minor arrhythmias), milk thistle (liver disease), turmeric (rheumatoid arthritis), and uva ursi (urinary tract infections).

Many other alternative approaches are also achieving increased acceptance. Chiropractic, visualizations, acupuncture, and massage are some of the more prominent.

What This Means for the Future of Alternative Medicine

Up until the last several years, alternative medicine has endured (and sometimes enjoyed) the position of outsider. It has lacked general respectability, funding, and all the other perquisites of status. In fact, powerful conventional medical institutions have endeavored quite religiously to stamp out or at least suppress alternative treatments. Conversely, alternative medicine has long utilized the prerogatives of the underdog to make reckless claims on behalf of its treatments and in criticism of conventional medicine.

If St. John's wort and other herbal treatments were ever to become accepted, however, alternative medicine would find itself on the brink of becoming mainstream. This would please certain elements and horrify others.

One strain in alternative medicine yearns for increasing scientific respectability. Bastyr University in Seattle is one institution that represents this wing, and many of its graduates are working hard to bring forward the scientific side of alternative medicine. They review formal research evidence, make use of cutting edge biochemistry, and propose and conduct scientific trials of their own.

But there is another large segment of alternative medicine that does not wish to join the scientific bandwagon. Practitioners in this camp favor the intuitive, fuzzy, subjective aspects of healing. In their view, as soon as a treatment becomes scientifically respectable, it ceases to be a truly alternative treatment and joins the mechanical, dehumanized, "left-brain" culture of conventional medicine. They prefer to function in a realm where gut feelings, intuitive sensibilities, and subjective talents can hold full sway.

These proponents of the right-brain approach will not be the only naysayers. There is also a strong rebellious strain in alternative medicine that instinctively doubts whatever conventional medicine accepts, no matter how humane, simply because conventional medicine accepts it, and prefers any treatment, no matter how technological, that conventional medicine opposes. Many advocates of alternative intravenous therapies fit into this group. If St. John's wort were to become an approved drug, such people would soon find strong reasons for disapproving of it!

Finally, alternative medicine also caters to the desire for simplistic, miraculous cures. This desire will never die, even if it is never fulfilled. Any responsible evaluation of treatment efficacy will always come up short from this perspective.

For all these reasons, certain facets of alternative treatment are destined to remain outside mainstream medicine. But with its combination of traditional usage and modern scientific verification, St. John's wort may help lead the way toward a partial rapprochement between conventional and alternative medicine.

Appendix:
Summary of the Research Record for St. John's Wort

Standardized extracts of St. John's wort have been widely investigated in Germany as treatment for mild to moderate depression (HAM-D scores under 25). Probably the best designed study was performed in 1993 by the German physician K. D. Hansgen and his colleagues.[1] In this four-week trial, seventy-two moderately depressed patients from eleven different physicians' practices were selected based on *DSM III* criteria for major depression. They were then randomized into two groups: one that received placebos and another that received 300 milligrams three times a day of an extract of St. John's wort standardized to contain 0.3 percent hypericin.

Initial HAM-D scores averaged 21.8 in the St. John's wort group. By four weeks they had fallen to 9.2. In the placebo group, HAM-D scores dropped only half as much, yielding a statistically significant difference ($p < .001$). Over 80 percent of the patients taking St. John's wort improved significantly (greater than 50 percent drop in HAM-D scores), while only 26 percent of the placebo group responded. There were five dropouts, primarily due to worsening of depression in the placebo group.

An additional thirty-six patients were added to the trial in 1996, and the study methodology was repeated.[2] The results followed the same pattern as before.

In the remaining St. John's wort studies, older ICD-9 criteria for depression were used. Otherwise, protocols were similar.

In one study, the effectiveness of St. John's wort was evaluated in 105 mildly depressed patients (average HAM-D of about 16) drawn from three physicians' practices.[3] At the end of the four-week trial, 67 percent of the patients on St. John's wort showed satisfactory response to treatment (greater than 50 percent reduction in HAM-D scores), compared to only 28 percent of those patients on placebo. Significant improvements were particularly noted in mood, anxiety, and insomnia.

One of the longest studies on St. John's wort was performed in 1991. It followed fifty patients for eight weeks, and once more the herb proved significantly more effective than placebo.[4] Yet another multicenter study performed in 1991 showed positive results in 116 patients followed for six weeks.[5] However, this study suffered from one significant drawback: the St. John's wort was administered in the form of drops, which may have been distinguishable from placebo based on taste.

Altogether, there have been fourteen St. John's wort versus placebo randomized double-blind studies.[6] In 1995, E. Ernst published a criteria-based review of the literature and narrowed the field down to nine St. John's wort versus placebo studies involving 635 patients.[7] The cumulative results make a compelling case that St. John's wort is an effective treatment for depression.

Six trials have compared St. John's wort against tricyclic antidepressants. Unfortunately, these were all flawed because they used subtherapeutic doses of the comparator.

Mechanism

The mechanism of action of St. John's wort remains unknown.

Early research showed that extracts of St. John's wort can inhibit the enzyme monoamine-oxidase in vitro.[8] Later investigation demonstrated, however, that the dosages of St. John's wort taken orally in actual practice are probably far too low to inhibit monoamine-oxidase in vivo.[9] As noted below, MAO-inhibitor-type reactions have never been observed with St. John's wort.

More recent research has focused on serotonin. In one study, investigators observed that St. John's wort extract suppressed the expression of serotonin receptors in neuroblastoma cells.[10] Another study noted elevations of serotonin and dopamine levels in the brains of rats and mice fed St. John's wort extracts.[11]

Side Effects

In the extensive German experience with St. John's wort as a treatment for depression, there have been no published reports of serious adverse consequences.[12] In particular, no MAO inhibitor-type reactions have ever been reported.

In an open drug-monitoring study of 3,250 patients taking St. John's wort extract for four weeks, the overall incidence of side effects was 2.4 percent.[13] The most common were mild stomach discomfort (0.6 percent), allergic reactions (0.5 percent), tiredness (0.4 percent), and restlessness (0.3 percent). Only 1.5 percent of the patients dropped out of the study due to adverse reactions.

The overall incidence of side effects in the double-blind studies that compared St. John's wort against placebo was 4.1 percent.[14] However, studies that compared the effectiveness of St. John's wort against tricyclic drugs reported a much higher incidence of side effects, as did those using preparations combining St. John's wort with other herbs. It is the aberrant results of these studies that have given rise to a sometimes quoted side-effect rate of 19.8 percent.[15] This figure should be regarded as inflated.

Photosensitivity has occurred in animals that graze on St. John's wort. However, this side effect has never been reported among humans taking oral St. John's wort.[16]

Notes

1. Hansgen, K. D., et al. 1994. Multicenter double-blind study examining the antidepressant effectiveness of the hypericum extract LI 160. *Journal of Geriatric Psychiatry and Neurology* 7 (suppl. 1), S15–S18.

2. Hansgen, K. D., et al. 1996. Antidepressive Wirksamkeit eines hochdosierten Hypericum-Extraktes. *Munch. Med. Wschr.* 138, 35–39.

3. Harrer, G., et al. 1994. Placebo-controlled double-blind study examining the effectiveness of an hypericum preparation in 105 mildly de-

pressed patients. *Journal of Geriatric Psychiatry and Neurology* 7 (suppl. 1), S9–S11.

4. Reh, C., et al. 1992. Hypericum—Extrakt bel Depressionen—eine wirksame. *Alternative Therapiewoche* 42, 1576–1581.

5. Harrer, G., et al. 1991. "Alternative" Depressionsbehandlung mit einem Hypericum-Extrakt. *Therapiewoche Neurologie/Psychiatrie* 5, S710–S716.

6. Linde, K., et al. 1996. St. John's wort for depression: An overview and meta-analysis of randomised clinical trials. *British Medical Journal* 313, 253–258.

7. Ernst, E., 1995. St. John's wort, an anti-depressant? A systematic, criteria-based review. *Phytomedicine* 2 (1), 67–71.

8. Suzuki, O., et al. 1984. Inhibition of monamine oxidase by hypericin. *Planta Medica* 50, 2722–2724.

9. Bladt, S., et al. 1994. Inhibition of MAO by fractions and constituents of hypericum extract. *Journal of Geriatric Psychiatry and Neurology* 7 (suppl. 1), S57–S59.

10. Muller, W. E. G., et al. 1994. Effects of hypericum extract on the expression of serotonin receptors. *Journal of Geriatric Psychiatry and Neurology* 7 (suppl. 1), S63–S64.

11. Winterhoff, H., et al. 1993. Pharmacological screening of hypericum perforatum L. in animals. *Nervenheilkunde* 12, 341–345.

12. Smet, P., and Nolen, W. 1996. St. John's wort as an anti-depressant. *British Medical Journal* 3, 241–242.

13. Woelk, H., et al. 1994. Benefits and risks of the hypericum extract LI 160: Drug monitoring study with 3250 patients. *Journal of Geriatric Psychiatry and Neurology* 7 (suppl. 1), S34–S38.

14. Linde, K., et al. 1996.

15. Ibid., p. 253.

16. Seigers, C. P., et al. 1993. Phototoxicity caused by hypericum. *Nervenheilkunde* 12, 320–322.

Notes

1. Balon, R., et al. 1993. Sexual dysfunction during antidepressant treatment. *Journal of Clinical Psychiatry* 54, 209–212.

2. Linde, K., et al. 1996. St. John's wort for depression: An overview and meta-analysis of randomised clinical trials. *British Medical Journal* 313, 253–258.

3. American Medical Association. 1990. *Drug Evaluation Subscription* 1, 1–13.

4. Hansgen, K. D., et al. 1994. Multicenter double-blind study examining the antidepressant effectiveness of the hypericum extract LI 160. *Journal of Geriatric Psychiatry and Neurology* 7 (suppl. 1), S15–S18.

5. Hansgen, K. D., et al. 1996. Antidepressive Wirksamkeit eines hochdosierten Hypericum-Extraktes. *Munch. Med. Wschr.* 138, 35–39.

6. Harrer, G., et al. 1994. Placebo-controlled double-blind study examining the effectiveness of an hypericum preparation in 105 mildly depressed patients. *Journal of Geriatric Psychiatry and Neurology* 7 (suppl. 1), S9–S11.

7. Reh, C., et al. 1992. Hypericum—Extrakt bel Depressionen—eine wirksame. *Alternative Therapiewoche* 42, 1576–1581.

8. Harrer, G., et al. 1991. "Alternative" Depressionsbehandlung mit einem Hypericum-Extrakt. *Therapiewoche Neurologie Psychiatre* 5, S710–S716.

9. Ernst, E. 1995. St. John's wort, an anti-depressant? A systematic, criteria-based review. *Phytomedicine* 2 (1), 67–71.

10. Linde, K., et al. 1996.

11. Smet, P., and Nolen, W. 1996. St. John's wort as an anti-depressant. *British Medical Journal* 3, 241–242.

12. *Physician's Desk Reference* (p. 938). 1997. Montvale, N.J.: Medical Economics Company, Inc.

13. Suzuki, O., et al. 1984. Inhibition of monamine oxidase by hypericin. *Planta Medica* 50, 272–274.

14. Bladt, S., et al. 1994. Inhibition of MAO by fractions and constituents of hypericum extract. *Journal of Geriatric Psychiatry and Neurology* 7 (suppl. 1), S57–S59.

15. Muller, W. E. G., et al. 1994. Effects of hypericum extract on the expression of serotonin receptors. *Journal of Geriatric Psychiatry and Neurology* 7 (suppl. 1), S63–S64.

16. Winterhoff, H., et al. 1993. Pharmacological screening of hypericum perforatum L. in animals. *Nervenheilkunde* 12, 341–345.

17. Smet, P., and Nolen, W. 1996.

18. Woelk, H., et al. 1994. Benefits and risks of the hypericum extract LI 160: Drug monitoring study with 3250 patients. *Journal of Geriatric Psychiatry and Neurology* 7 (suppl. 1), S34–S38.

19. Linde, K., et al. 1996.

20. Ibid., 253–258.

21. *Physician's Desk Reference* (p. 936). 1997. Montvale, N.J.: Medical Economics Company, Inc.

22. Smet, P., and Nolen, W. 1996.

23. Seigers, C. P., et al. 1993. Phototoxicity caused by hypericum. *Nervenheilkunde* 12, 320–322.

24. Mcauliffe, V., et al. 1993. A phase I dose escalation study of synthetic hypericin in HIV infected patients. *National Conference Human Retroviruses Related to Infection* (1 st), 159.

25. Linde, K., et al. 1996.

26. Smet, P., and Nolen, W. 1996.

27. Weiss, R. F. 1988. *Herbal Medicine* (pp. 295–297), translated by A. R. Meuss. England: Beaconsfield Publishers Ltd.

28. Kreitsch, K., et al. 1988. Prevalence, presenting symptoms, and psychological characteristics of individuals experiencing a diet-related mood disturbance. *Behav. Ther.* 19, 593–604.

29. Vorbach, E. V., et al. 1994. Effectiveness and tolerance of the hypericum extract LI 160 in comparison with imipramine: Randomized double-blind study with 135 outpatients. *Journal of Geriatric Psychiatry and Neurology* 7 (suppl. 1), S19–S23.

30. Thase, M., et al. 1996. A placebo-controlled, randomized clinical trial comparing sertraline and imipramine for the treatment of dysthymia. *Archives of General Psychiatry* 53 (9), 777–784.

31. Harrer, G., et al. 1994. Effectiveness and tolerance of the hypericum extract LI 160 compared to maprotiline: A multicenter double-blind study. *Journal of Geriatric Psychiatry and Neurology* 7 (suppl. 1), S24–S28.

32. Smet, P., and Nolen, W. 1996.

33. Dunlop, S. R., et al. 1990. Pattern analysis shows beneficial effect of fluoxetine treatment in mild depression. *Psychopharmacology Bulletin* 26, 173–180.

34. Harrer, G., et al. 1994, S9–S11.

35. Thase, M., et al. 1996.

36. Stewart, J. W., et al. 1985. Treatment outcome validation of DSM-II depressive subtypes. *Archives of General Psychiatry* 42, 1148–1153.

37. Linde, K., et al. 1996.

38. Weiss, R. F., 1988. *Herbal Medicine* (p. 228) edited by A. R Meuss. England: Beaconsfield Publishers Ltd.

39. Greenberg, R. P., et al. 1994. A meta-analysis of fluoxetine outcome in the treatment of depression. *Journal of Nervous and Mental Diseases* 182 (10), 547–551.

40. Woelk, H., et al. 1994.

41. Linde, K., et al. 1996.

42. Balon, R., et al. 1993.

43. Linden, J., et al. 1992. Fluoxetin in der Anwendung durch niedergelassene Nervenarzte. *Munch. Med. Wschr.* 134, 836–840.

44. Stokes, P. E. 1993. Fluoxetine: A five-year review. *Clinical Therapeutics* 15 (2), 216–243.

45. Ibid.

46. Vorbach, E. V., et al. 1994.

47. Thase, M., et al. 1996.

48. Harrer, G., et al. 1994, S24–S28; Vorbach, E. V. 1994.

49. Katon, W. 1987. The epidemiology of depression in medical care. *Int. J. Psychiatry Med.* 17, 93–112.

50. Broadhead, W. E., et al. 1990. Depression, disability days, and days lost from work in a prospective epidemiologic survey. *JAMA* 264, 2524–2528.

51. Wells, K. B., et al. 1989. The functioning and well-being of depressed patients: Results from the medical outcomes study. *JAMA* 262, 914–919.

52. Hubner, W. D., et al. 1994. Hypericum treatment of mild depressions with somatic symptoms. *Journal of Geriatric Psychiatry and Neurology* 7 (suppl. 1), S12–S14.

53. Linde, K., et al. 1996.

54. Hansgen, K. D., et al. 1994.

55. Woelk, H., et al. 1994.

56. Murray, M. 1995. *The Healing Power of Herbs: The Enlightened Person's Guide to the Wonders of Medicinal Plants* (p. 145). Rocklin: Prima Publishing.

57. Eckmann, F. 1990. Cerebral insufficiency treatment with ginkgo-biloba extract: Time of onset of effect in a double-blind study with 60 inpatients. *Fortschr. Med.* 108, 557–560.

58. Schubert, H., et al. 1993. Depressive episode primarily unresponsive to therapy in elderly patients: Efficacy of ginkgo-biloba (Egb 761) in combination with antidepressants. *Geriatr. Forsch.* 3, 45–53.

59. Huguet, F., et al. 1994. Decreased cerebral 5-HT receptors during aging: Reversal by ginkgo-biloba extract (Egb 761). *J. Pharm. Pharmacol.* 46, 316–318.

60. Murray, M. 1995.

61. Heller, B. 1978. Pharmacological and clinical effects of D-phenylalanine in depression and Parkinson's disease. In *Noncatecholic Phenylethylamines, Part 1* (pp. 397–417), edited by Mosnaim and Wolf. New York: Marcel Dekker.

62. Beckmann H., et al. 1979. DL-phenylalanine versus imipramine: A double-blind controlled study. *Arch. Psychiat. Nervenkr.* 227, 49–58. See also Beckmann, H. 1983. Phenylalanine in affective disorders. *Adv. Biol. Psychiatry* 10, 137–147.

63. Cenachi, T., et al. 1993. Cognitive decline in the elderly: A double-blind, placebo-controlled multicenter study on efficacy of phosphatidyl serine administration. *Aging* 5, 123–133.

64. Ibid.

65. Maggioni, M., et al. 1990. Effects of phosphatidylserine therapy in geriatric patients with depressive disorders. *Acta Psychiatr. Scand.* 81, 265–270.

66. Werbach, M. 1991. *Nutritional Influences on Mental Illness* (pp. 255–271). Tarzana, CA: Third Line Press.

67. Bratman, S. 1997. *The Alternative Medicine Sourcebook: A Realistic Evaluation of Alternative Healing Methods* (pp. 93–94). Los Angeles: Lowell House.

68. Kinzler, E., et al. 1991. Clinical efficacy of a kava extract in patients with anxiety syndrome: Double-blind placebo controlled study over 4 weeks. *Arzneim. Forsch.* 41, 584–588.

69. Munte, T. F., et al. 1993. Effects of oxazepam and an extract of kava roots (piper methysticum) on event-related potentials in a word recognition task. *Neuropsychobiol.* 27, 46–53.

70. Mathews, J. D., et al. 1988. Effects of the heavy usage of kava on physical health: Summary of a pilot survey in an Aboriginal community. *Med. J. Aust.* 148, 548–555.

71. Lindahl, O., et al. 1989. Double-blind study of a valerian preparation. *Pharmacol. Biochem. Behav.* 432 (4), 1065–1066. Leathwood, P. D., et al. 1985. Aqueous extract of valerian reduces latency to fall asleep in man. *Planta Medica* 54, 144–148.

Index

Index

Stress, Anxiety & Insomnia

How You Can Benefit from Diet, Vitamins, Minerals, Herbs, and Exercise

Michael T. Murray, N.D.

ISBN 1-55958-489-0 / paperback / 192 pages
U.S. $11.00 / Can. $14.95

You can relieve stress, anxiety, insomnia, and similar problems without, resorting to dangerous drugs and chemicals to do it. A leading researcher in naturopathic medicine shows how in this helpful, reassuring book. With Dr. Michael T. Murray's thoughtful, comprehensive approach, you will learn how to use simple exercise routines, natural foods, and plant-based remedies to:

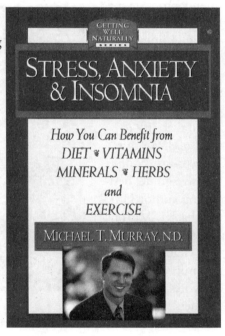

- Relax and reduce anxiety
- Help your body fight stress
- Fall asleep without artificial aids
- Improve your overall health
- And much more

This important book can change your life!

Encyclopedia of Nutritional Supplements

The Essential Guide for Improving Your Health Naturally

Michael T. Murray, N.D.

ISBN 0-7615-0410-9 / paperback / 576 pages
U.S. $19.95 / Can. $26.95

Nutritional supplements promote overall health and well-being, minimize the effects of aging, strengthen the immune system, and encourage the body's natural ability to heal itself. In this easy-to-use, comprehensive guide, best-selling author Dr. Michael T. Murray introduces you to key vitamins, minerals, nutrients, oils, enzymes, and extracts. He

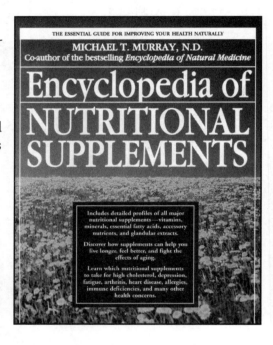

describes in detail the healing properties of each and explains symptoms that may indicate a deficiency. Most important, he details the health conditions that each supplement can improve. With recommendations for use and dosage, this essential healing resource gives you the power to improve your health naturally.